Dedication

Grace Abelson DeFries
1890-1985

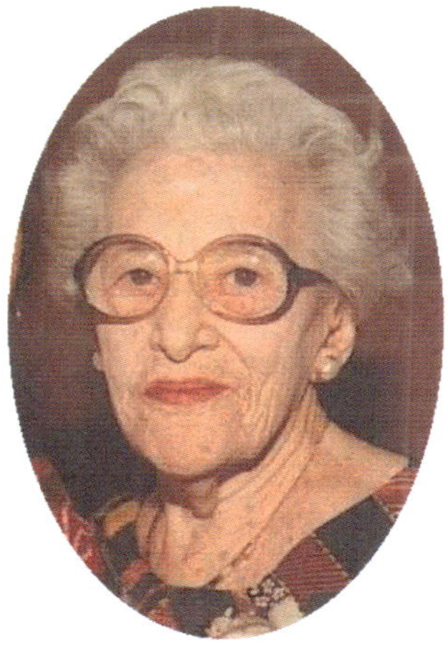

Grace Abelson DeFries was blessed with a long and eventful life devoted to the well-being of her family and community. Her grandchildren remember her visits as always generating a trail of fresh baked pies, stacks of blintzes and gifts of hand-knitted sweaters and afghans. Even after her hands were gnarled with arthritis and her hearing was gone, she retained a composure that belied all her hard work. She was never too busy to listen, to understand and to accept. Her three granddaughters lovingly remember her as Grandma Sugarplum, for that was the name she lovingly called each of them.

She gradually lost almost all hearing over the last years of her life. Only grudgingly did she seek the help of hearing aids and a few assistive devices. Her fierce independence and desire to hide all deficiencies by denial undoubtedly limited the utility she was able to derive from them, although the devices of those days left much to be desired.

Grace Abelson DeFries passed away at the age of 95. Her son and grandchildren dedicate this guide to those who are struggling with advancing hearing loss. We sincerely hope that it will be of assistance and help ease their problems.

Mike, Diane, Vicki, and Ruth DeFries

"I Can't Hear You!" was compiled and edited by the Northern Virginia Resource Center for Deaf and Hard of Hearing Persons (NVRC) with the generous support of the Grace Abelson DeFries Memorial Fund (GADMF).

NVRC's mission is *to empower deaf and hard of hearing individuals through education, advocacy and community involvement.* The Center was established in 1987 to serve the Northern Virginia area and has achieved national recognition as one of the top centers for deaf and hard of hearing people in the U.S.

The GADMF was established at NVRC in 2005 by Mike DeFries and family to assist the Center in its outreach efforts. The fund is targeted to supporting those who experience hearing loss as they age, to enable them to cope and thrive. We hope it will also educate their families and caregivers about the physical and emotional impact of hearing loss.

The GADMF is thankful to Bonnie O'Leary, coordinator and editor of this guide; to Melody Hotek for its "artistic" conception and composition; to Cheryl Heppner, Executive Director of NVRC; and to all others who worked tirelessly to produce this publication.

GADMF and NVRC are thankful to Dr. Neil Bauman, GuidePost Publications, for his invaluable assistance in the printing of this book.

3951 Pender Drive, Suite 130, Fairfax, Virginia 22030
703-352-9055 (V), 9056 (TTY), 9058 (Fax)
www.nvrc.org info@nvrc.org

First printing April, 2009

The origin of the cat on the cover remains a mystery, but we did find it on the Internet in a blog by Cole, WXYC, Chapel Hill, NC. Cole, if this was your photo, many thanks.

***Ray Scheid, Cartoonist**, is a retired artist-illustrator with 30 years of Federal service working for the U.S. Navy in Washington, D.C. He lost his hearing in 1964.*

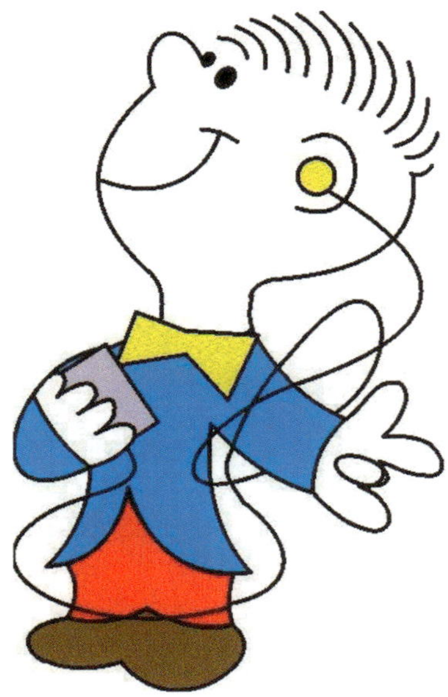

"Little Raymo"
© Ray Scheid

Table of Contents

Introduction

Dear Friends,

The process of creating "I Can't Hear You!" was a labor of love by a very enthusiastic group of people. We were united in our determination to provide a variety of helpful information to individuals who have late-onset hearing loss, and to their families, friends and caregivers.

We wrote this booklet with the intention that it be both easy to follow and fun to read. You won't find a detailed discussion of various medical conditions or drugs that can cause hearing loss, the many uses of captioning, or all the different kinds of hearing assistive technology. A lot of additional material simply couldn't be incorporated due to space constraints. We would have ended up with an encyclopedia!

We hope that this booklet will whet your appetite and motivate you to get in touch with the Northern Virginia Resource Center for Deaf and Hard of Hearing Persons to learn more or be directed to our best information sources. You'll find a bit about our Center's services on page 60, and our contact information is inside the front cover.

Often the most useful information on coping with the loss of hearing is not from professionals but from others who have experienced its impact. We were fortunate to find many individuals with wisdom and hindsight who were generous in sharing their talents for the articles in this booklet so it could truly be written "by the people, for the people." We hope that you will enjoy their contributions to these pages.

Happy reading!

Warmly,
Cheryl

NVRC

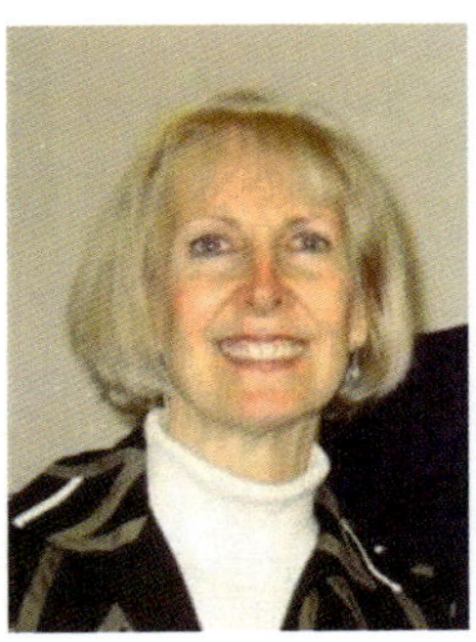

***Cheryl Heppner** became Executive Director of NVRC in January, 1991. Deafened by spinal meningitis shortly before her seventh birthday, Cheryl attended public school with hearing classmates and graduated with a degree in Journalism from Penn State. She voices, signs, speechreads, and is an avid user of assistive technology. Cheryl was a hearing aid wearer until February 2000, when she received a cochlear implant. She is a tireless advocate on national, state, regional and local levels, and has received numerous awards. Her articles are widely read in national journals.*

Preface
First Things First—Do I Have a Hearing Loss?

If you suspect you aren't hearing as well as you used to, chances are you're right — and you are not alone! An estimated 55 million Americans have some degree of hearing loss. It is a normal part of aging. Among seniors, it is the third most prevalent health condition after arthritis and hypertension, affecting one in three by age 65, and two in three by 75.

Now, how about you? What kinds of hearing difficulties are you experiencing? Are you struggling with any of these "top ten" early warning signs of hearing loss?

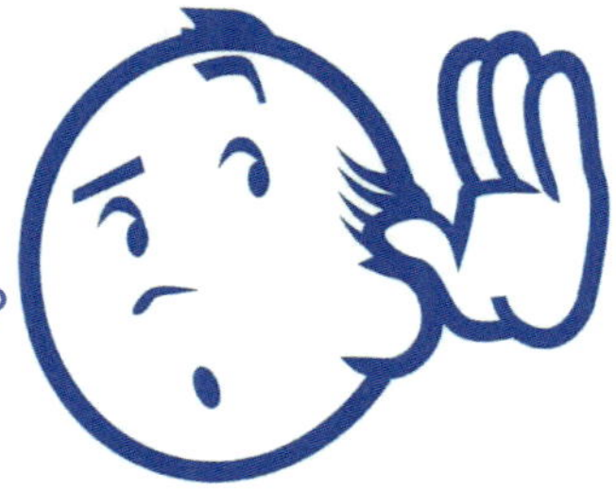

1. *Does it seem to you that people mumble most of the time?*
2. *Do you ask people to repeat what they are saying?*
3. *Are women's and children's voices harder for you to understand than men's?*
4. *Do people complain about the volume of your television?*
5. *Do you hear people speaking but have trouble understanding what they are saying?*
6. *Do you have ringing or other mysterious noises in your ears?*
7. *Is it hard for you to follow a conversation in a noisy environment?*
8. *Do you have trouble following dialog on TV, in the theatre, or at the movies?*
9. *Do your loved ones say you need a hearing test?*
10. *Are you spending less time socializing with friends and relatives than you would like?*

If you answered "yes" to any of these questions, chances are you could benefit from having your hearing evaluated by a professional to determine what type and how much of a hearing loss you have.

There are abundant resources for people with hearing loss today. We hope you find the information in this booklet to be helpful as you explore solutions that might work well for you.

Chapter One
Living and Laughing with Hearing Loss

By Bonnie O'Leary

During the hubbub of a recording session, a client asked me for a paper clip. After I handed it to him, he stared down at it quietly for a second, looked back up at me with a puzzled expression on his face, laughed, and said "CUP! Do you have a paper CUP!?"

I knew I was becoming hard of hearing at that time, but rather than do something about it, I had been diligently honing my skills at becoming Ms. Bonnie O'Bluff. That's what most of us do when we start to lose our hearing—we bluff our way over, around and through conversations, hoping that no one notices how many words are flying past us as verbal UFOs. I appreciated my client's immediate resolve to ease my twinge of embarrassment and laugh the moment away.

Learning to live and laugh with hearing loss takes time, patience, an understanding of the strategies we need to communicate more easily with others, and, particularly, a good sense of humor! Hearing loss doesn't seem funny at all when we are first confronted with it. Here we are, trying to blend in with the activities at hand, when all of a sudden we either say something that has no relevance to the discussion or react inappropriately to what is being said to us. Zing! Gotcha! No matter how good natured the little smirk or eyeball roll from our loved ones may be, we can still feel wounded. But I've discovered that my most effective coping strategy through the years has been finding humor in my miscommunications. I try to think of them as scenes from funny TV shows, and I ask myself, "what would Lucille Ball or Bob Hope have done with *that*?!"

I'd like to share two of my favorites. The first happened after I checked in for a large, "hoity toity" luncheon reception. The hostess followed me through the busy lobby and whispered something to me. "Oops!" I smiled at her as I spoke. "You're on my deaf side, I didn't hear what you said." She ran quickly to my other side and whispered something in that ear, but I had to tell her that I still couldn't understand because I was hard of hearing in that ear. So now, as I was surrounded by a crowd of very elegantly dressed reception guests, the hostess blurted out for all to hear, "I said YOU HAVE YOUR SWEATER ON INSIDE OUT!"

The second happened a few years ago but remains one of the most often-repeated miscommunication stories here at NVRC, providing great amusement at my community outreach programs. I answered a call at our office from a woman who explained that she had an appointment to bring her mother in that Friday and needed directions to our location. I provided her with the directions and then asked what her mother was interested in trying out so we could have it ready for her. Was it a PockeTalker? an amplified phone? a television listening system? After a brief but awkward silence, the woman realized she had the wrong number. "Oh, I'm sorry," she apologized, "I thought I was calling Meineke. I have an appointment to bring my *muffler* in on Friday!"

I have many friends who don't hear well, and when we socialize we often swap miscommunication stories and laugh together. Using humor has enormous healing power for us. It helps us look past the reaction we sometimes get from hearing people when we misunderstand what they say and focus instead on how absurd or hilarious that misunderstanding actually is. In many ways, it helps us accept our own hearing losses from a more agreeable perspective. Many of us took speechreading classes with Dr. Scott Bally, whose articles appear on pages 47 and 51. Dr. Bally's use of humor in our classes helped break the ice for those who were new to hearing loss, and gave us all a foundation for our shared experiences.

When I was a hearing person, I used to own a recording studio. One of our clients was a gospel group, and when their album was finished I took a cassette copy to play in the car. My daughter, who was 12 at the time and had perfect hearing, thought this group was fantastic. Every time we drove anywhere she would ask if we could listen to the tape. The refrain of her favorite number started with the lyrics "oh, give me that old redemption power!", and one day she starting belting out with great zest and feeling, "oh, give me that old gray denture powder!" So you see, even the most perfect ears can miss those verbal UFOs!

I enjoy the Reader's Digest. I always read the "Laughter is the Best Medicine" section before anything else; there are so many opportunities in every day life to find the humor in a situation. Now that I have such a substantial hearing loss, I seem to be creating these situations around me all the time. And I've learned a neat trick. If I misunderstand someone, I'll ask him or her to rephrase what was said so I can make some sense of it. Then I will repeat what I *thought* was said the first time around. If he or she laughs, I laugh. Sometimes the person will say "that's a good one! I'll have to remember that one!" and I realize how far I've come to acknowledge and accept the lighter side of my hearing loss. More importantly, I'm able to share it with anyone who will listen. In doing so, I'm educating others about hearing loss in a way that they will remember with a smile and a warm heart.

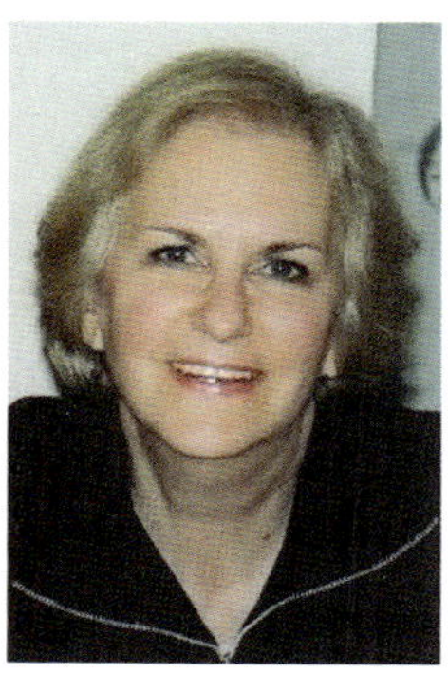

***Bonnie O'Leary** has been working with the NVRC since January 2002, focusing on outreach to senior citizens who have hearing loss and education for hearing families, caregivers and supervisors. She received her certification as a Hearing Loss Support Specialist and Peer Mentor from Gallaudet University in 2007. As a late-deafened adult, Bonnie applies her own personal experience with hearing loss to her outreach work. During her "hearing" years, Bonnie worked in advertising in New York and London and owned a 24-track recording studio in Burke, Virginia.*

Chapter Two
The Miraculous Journey of Sound

Our Amazing Ears—Listen Up!

In order to understand our hearing loss, it helps to know how the ear works. It's a highly complex organ which governs our balance as well as our hearing. As you can see from the simplified diagram on page 4, the ear is divided into three parts:

The Outer Ear

The outer ear is comprised of the part of the ear that we can see, known as the *pinna*, along with the part that the doctor sees when he or she looks into our ear, known as the ear canal. The *pinna* not only holds up our eyeglasses and shows off our earrings, it also functions as a baseball catcher's mitt, catching sounds in the air and funneling them into the ear canal. The ear canal senses the vibrations of the sound and passes them along to the eardrum. Most of us are familiar with the ear canal, especially those of us who have had "swimmer's ear" or problems with wax build-up. And whenever we're tempted to use that Q-Tip, we remember the doctor's warning: "Never put anything smaller than your elbow into your ear canal!"

The Middle Ear

The eardrum sits at the end of the ear canal, separating the outer ear from the middle ear. The middle ear is a chamber filled with air. It houses the three tiniest bones in the body called *ossicles*: the *malleus,* the *incus,* and the *stapes*. These tiny bones form a lever system connecting the eardrum to the inner ear. The little lever system is set in motion when the eardrum vibrates. Sounds that have been caught by the *pinna* and funneled through the ear canal are now amplified in this echo chamber before continuing to the inner ear.

The Inner Ear

The inner ear houses the *cochlea*, a snail-like bone structure that's lined with membranes and filled with fluid and thousands of tiny sensory (hair) cells. When we are born, each of these hair cells has already been programmed to respond to specific high, mid-range or low pitch sounds that we hear every day. Sounds are then transformed into electric impulses, passed to the *auditory nerve* and carried to *auditory cortex* in the brain, which then identifies the sound. That's right! We hear with our brain, not with our ears!

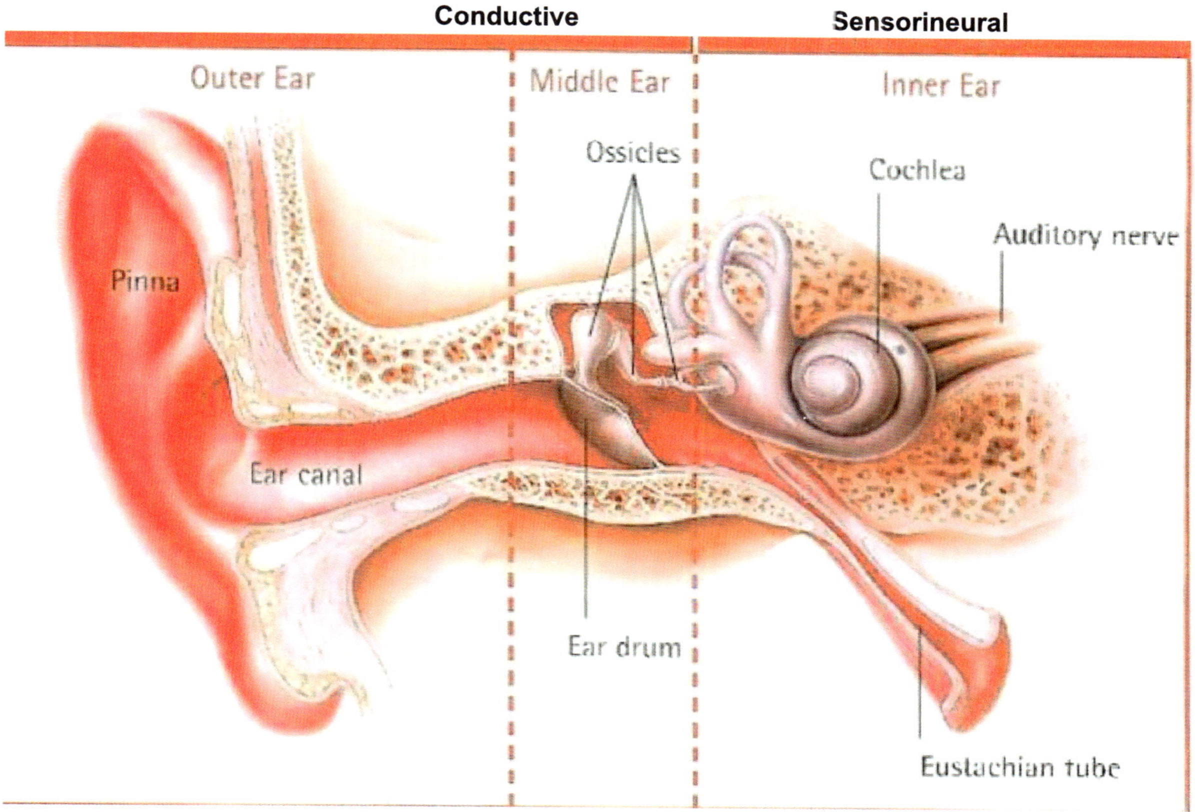

Reprinted from "EduLink," a publication for PHONAK hearing systems

Types and Causes of Hearing Loss

There are three types of hearing loss: *conductive*, *sensorineural*, and *mixed*.

Conductive hearing loss occurs when a problem in the outer and/or middle ear blocks the sound from reaching the inner ear. Causes of conductive hearing loss include a build-up of excess wax or other obstructions in the ear canal, holes in the eardrum, fluid in the middle ear, bony growths on the *ossicles*, or various ear infections. Most of the time, conductive hearing loss can be remedied by medical intervention.

Sensorineural hearing loss is the most common and is associated with changes in the cochlea or the auditory nerve. As we age, the little hair cells in the cochlea become inactive and do not regenerate. Causes of this type of hearing loss include genetics, prolonged exposure to noise, head trauma, illness, autoimmune disorders, certain medications, and tumors. Hearing loss in seniors is referred to as "*presbycusis*."

Mixed hearing loss is a combination of both *conductive* and *sensorineural*.

It is very important to **see your doctor** just to be sure there are no underlying medical problems causing your hearing loss. Doctors who treat ears are known as Otolaryngologists, or Ear, Nose and Throat specialists. Your doctor will tell you if you should make an appointment with an audiologist or hearing aid specialist.

Tinnitus

If you have ringing in your ears, you are not hallucinating! This "phantom" sound, known as *tinnitus**, is very real and very exasperating. The name tinnitus is from the Latin word meaning "to tinkle or to ring like a bell." But some sufferers might call it "buzzitus," "screechitus," "chirpitus," "whooshitus" or "hummmmmmmitus." Often referred to as a "bedeviling condition," tinnitus has been driving people crazy for centuries. The exact cause is still unknown and there is still no known cure.

Tinnitus may come from damaged hair cells in the cochlea. These hair cells are constantly firing off electrical impulses because they perceive that a sound is present even when it is not. It may be triggered or made worse by a variety of conditions. These include loud noises; ear infections; noise-induced hearing loss; wax build-up; jaw misalignment; certain medications; head and neck trauma; tumors on the auditory, vestibular or facial nerves; and cardiovascular disease. Sometimes, in some people, the intensity of the tinnitus will abate if these underlying conditions are treated.

Some sufferers have reported varying degrees of success with the use of hearing aids, cochlear implants, relaxation techniques, and alternative methods such as magnets and hypnosis. Cognitive therapies have also been known to help treat the emotional reaction to having tinnitus, and for some people the use of masking techniques has been effective. Many people who have tinnitus agree that they aren't as aware of it when they're busy and distracted by activities. It's more apparent and more frustrating during quiet times or at night, at bedtime. Masking noises include recorded sounds such as the ocean, thunderstorms, other "nature" sounds, or music that can be turned on at bedtime to help cope with tinnitus at the end of the day.

Tinnitus Retraining Therapy involves counseling and the use of ear-level or desk-top noise generators which help retrain the brain not to focus on the tinnitus.

Salt, caffeine, alcohol, sugar, fatigue and stress have been implicated in making tinnitus worse, but scientific studies do not consistently support this.

*Tinnitus is pronounced either ti-NIGHT-us or TIN-i-tus. They are both correct but ti-NIGHT-us is used by the American Tinnitus Association. For more information, contact the American Tinnitus Association, 65 SW Yamhill St., Suite 200, Portland, OR 97204. 1-800-634-8978. www.ata.org.

AMERICAN TINNITUS ASSOCIATION

Ode to Tinnitus

By Tonilyn Todd
(A.K.A. Cassie)

Crickets, dear crickets,
Get out of my ear.
I like you a lot,
But not always that near.

You buzz and you hum,
You make lots of noise.
But when u cover voices,
I can't keep my poise.

I stumble in conversations,
I say "Huh?" a lot.
I comment inappropriately,
You always put me on the spot!

So crickets, dear crickets,
Get out of my head,
I'm not usually cruel,
But I wish you were dead!

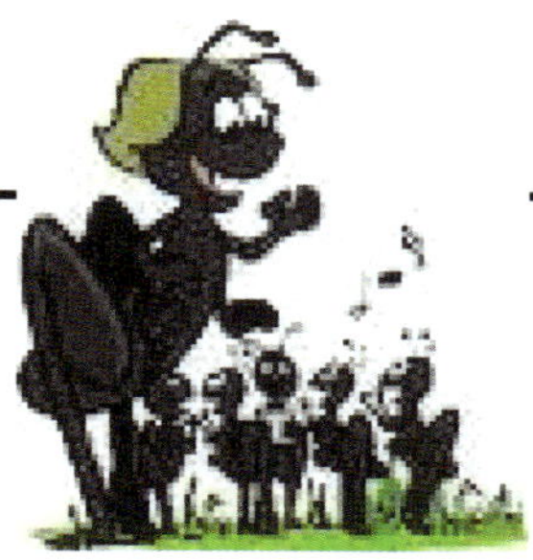

Tonilyn Todd *grew up hard of hearing and is now deaf, due to Meniere's Disease. She is also a brain tumor survivor, has low vision and is considered deaf-blind. That hasn't slowed her down, though. Tonilyn has an Associate's degree and enjoys drawing, writing, reading, computers, and learning languages/writing systems.*

Reprinted with permission from ALDA Reader 2005 (Association of Late-Deafened Adults)

In the Navy

By Dana Gumb

I was in the Navy in the 1940s aboard a light cruiser. My specialty was to operate the radar tracking equipment in the gun director mount which controlled the directional positioning of a dual five-inch gun mount located at deck level. The gun director is located at an upper level forward.

To prevent the five-inch gun mount from firing on its own director, a mechanical stop is located on the ship's deck. Unfortunately, on that day, the stop was not in place and the ship's firing mount actually fired on its own director. Fortunately, no one was killed, but I wound up with a loud ringing in the right ear – which still exists.

Medical professionals have told me to "live with it."

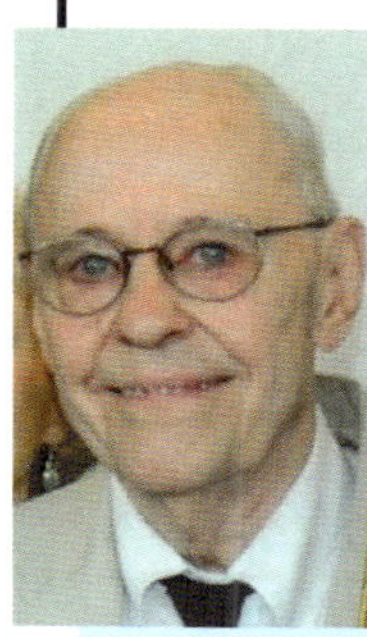

After six years in the Navy, ***Dana Gumb*** *resigned to the Naval Reserve and received a position in the Electronic Maintenance Office, Norfolk Naval Shipyard. Under the GI Bill, Dana received a Master's Degree from GA Tech, leading to employment with various electronic firms. In 1963, he was instrumental in establishing Vega Precision Laboratory to conceive, design, manufacture and field support aerospace electronic equipment. Mr. Gumb retired after 26 years.*

Chapter Three
"Techie" Stuff to the Rescue!

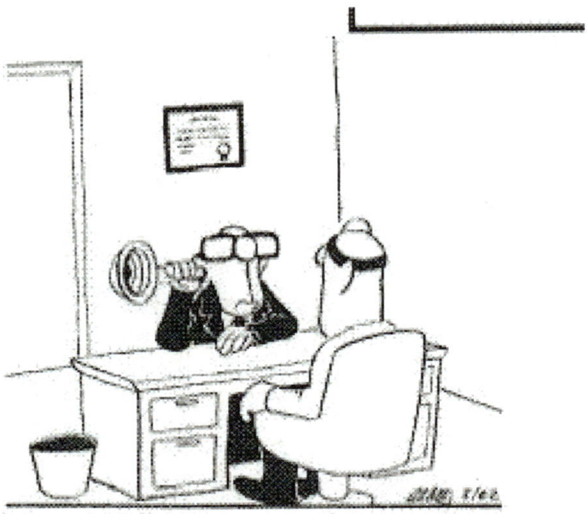

"I said, it's the only hearing aid covered by your insurance."

Hearing Aids

By Bonnie O'Leary

Welcome to the 21st century!

Today's hearing aids are made with a wide variety of circuitry options. Costs range from \$700 to \$3,200* per hearing aid, depending on the sophistication of the circuitry (details on the following pages!).

Medicare, most HMOs and private insurance will often pay <u>only</u> for the hearing tests, <u>not</u> the ear molds or hearing aids. (In some circumstances Medicaid will cover the cost of the aids.)

It's a good idea to check with your insurance company about the benefits before your evaluation. If coverage is provided, it might require you to see your doctor before buying the aid. To help you navigate the hearing aid journey, we've tried to simplify answers to some of the most frequently asked questions.

** prices as of Spring, 2009*

Audiologist or hearing aid dispenser? Who's who?

Audiologists are highly trained health care professionals. They are licensed by the state that regulates the scope of their practices. In addition to fitting and programming hearing aids, these professionals provide diagnostic services such as balance and dizziness evaluations, newborn infant screenings, and programming for cochlear implants. As of 2007, a doctorate (Au.D.) is the required graduate degree for becoming an audiologist. Audiologists who obtain an Au.D. are not physicians; they are Doctors of Audiology in the same way that optical specialists are Doctors of Optometry.

Hearing Aid Dealers must complete a certification course for fitting hearing aids and often learn while apprenticed to another dispenser. Each state has its own licensing requirements. Dealers develop expertise in hearing aid technology, fitting and programming, but do not make diagnostic evaluations, and often prefer to focus on one or two manufacturers of hearings aids, which can be limiting to the patient.

Where do I find a hearing health professional?

Word of mouth is a good start, but if you do not know anyone who has been successfully fitted with hearing aids, you can turn to a national resource such as the American Academy of Audiology which maintains a listing of professionals in your area. The Academy is located at 11730 Plaza America Dr., Suite 300, Reston, VA 20190. Phone number 1-800-222-2336, and web site http://www.audiology.org. Your doctor may also be able to provide a referral.

What are my options?

Will you want to continue to work with an independent professional as years go by or will you be more comfortable working with a group? Some audiologists team up with Ear, Nose and Throat (ENT) doctors as part of the same practice. An advantage to this arrangement is having your ENT and your audiologist under the same roof. A disadvantage is that when there's more than one audiologist, you might see a different audiologist than the one who fit your aids. The time allotted for an appointment may be shorter in some cases.

It is helpful to understand that some audiologists and dealers are under contract to sell a certain number of hearing aids per year, and that can influence their approach to your situation. In some cases, they might pressure you to buy because they are sales-driven, and this is not in your best interests. Other audiologists and dealers are more patient-driven, with genuine concern for creating better hearing for you. These professionals will put **you** before the sale, ensure that you have the time to adjust to your hearing aids and be willing to try another hearing aid manufacturer if the first one does not produce the desired result.

What are my rights?

The business part of the transaction is also important. Federal law requires dispensers to give patients a 30-day adjustment period to try out the hearing aids. Some audiologists allow 60 days. If at the end of the adjustment period you are not satisfied, regardless of the number of adjustments you have had, you can return the hearing aids for an exchange or a refund. Before you agree to buy the aid, be sure to ask about your audiologist's or dealer's refund policy. Some will charge as much as 20 percent of the cost of the hearing aids to return them; others will charge as little as 4 percent. If your hearing aids cost $5,000, return fees could range between $200 and $1,000!

Contact Info

Before committing to work with any hearing health professional, you may want to check with the Better Business Bureau for any registered complaints. The BBB is located at 1411 K Street NW, 10th Floor, Washington, DC 20005-3404. You can call 202-393-8000, go to http://www.dc.bbb.org, or contact your local branch.

What happens during a hearing evaluation?

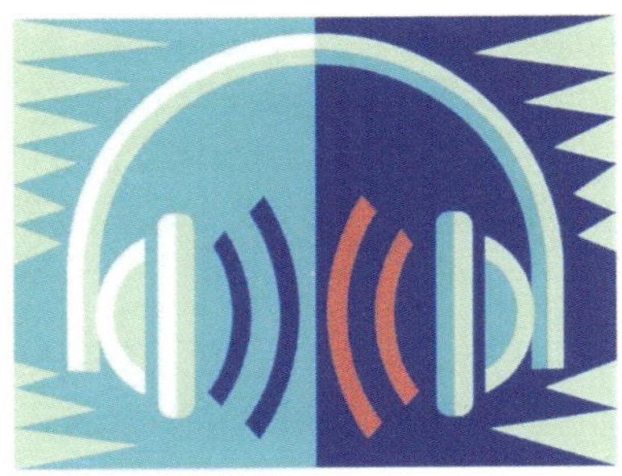

1. An interview by the hearing health professional

You'll talk about your overall health, any medications you take, when you noticed your hearing started to deteriorate, what types of listening situations are becoming challenging for you, and whether there are other considerations such as balance or vision problems, or manual dexterity difficulties caused by conditions such as arthritis that might hinder your ability to use the hearing aid control buttons or insert the batteries.

2. A physical examination of the ear

A physical examination of the ear with an otoscope (ear light) will be performed. This is painless and gives the hearing professional a look at your ear canal and eardrum to see if there are signs of wax build-up or other conditions that can be treated by a physician.

3. A hearing test using special headphones in a sound-proof booth

This test starts with pure tones presented to each ear individually. Pure tones are like the sound of a tuning fork— they range from low pitch to high pitch like the keys on a piano. The technical term for "pitch" is "frequency." When you hear a tone, you raise your hand or press a button to let the professional know you have heard it. Frequency is measured in Hertz (Hz).

The professional measures how soft a tone you can detect. This is called your pure tone threshold. The loudness or volume of the tone will vary, and some sounds will seem louder than others. The technical term for "volume" is "intensity," which is measured in decibels (dB).

The audiogram is a graph of the hearing test results. The professional marks an **O** for right ear and **X** for left ear. From the audiogram, you can see the pitches that had to be made louder in order for you to hear. You can also see if you have the same level of hearing loss in both ears. Your hearing loss will be categorized as mild, moderate, severe or profound. These categories relate to the degree of difficulty you may have hearing and understanding speech.

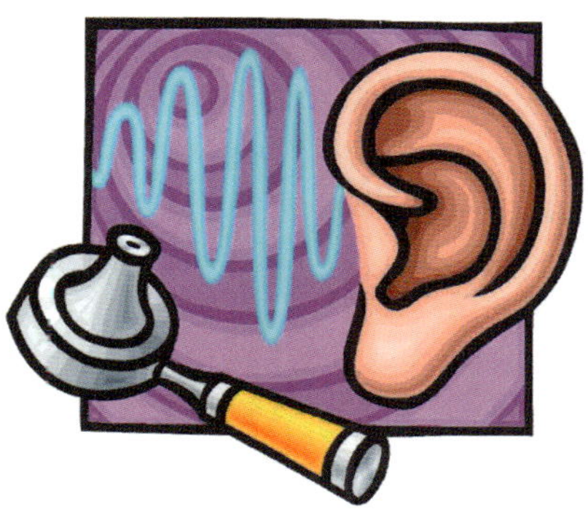

4. Speech recognition test

Speech recognition will be tested to determine how clearly you understand words when they are spoken at an adequate volume for your hearing loss. Your speech recognition scores are important measures for setting realistic expectations for the kind of improvement you may get with hearing aids.

5. Tympanograms may be recorded

A tympanogram will help determine if you have middle ear problems such as fluid in the ear, a hole in the eardrum or problems with the little bones in the middle ear. An airtight plug is inserted in the ear canal and the air pressure is changed slightly to test how well the ear drum moves with the change in pressure.

My audiogram confuses me! What does it mean?

All of the tests we have discussed will be recorded on an audiogram. You should be given a copy at the end of your session. Your hearing professional will go over the results of the tests with you and make recommendations for next steps if you have enough of a hearing loss to benefit from hearing aids.

Let's expand a bit on what you learned on page 10. Notice the numbers across the top of the audiogram; they represent the frequency of a sound, or the "pitch," which is measured in Hertz (Hz). The pitch goes from low (125 Hz) to high (8,000 Hz), or bass to treble, like the keys on a piano. Now look at the numbers going down the left side of the graph; these represent the volume or the sounds or intensity in decibels (dB). As you can see from the drawings, the louder sounds are towards the bottom of the audiogram.

Now look at the "X" near the picture of the piano. The X means that a 500 Hz tone had to be 80 dB in intensity for you to hear it in the left ear. You would still be able to hear a lawn mower humming, an airplane, some louder notes on the piano, and a jack hammer with that ear. You would have trouble hearing soft conversation and a baby's cry, and would be struggling to hear vowels and consonants.

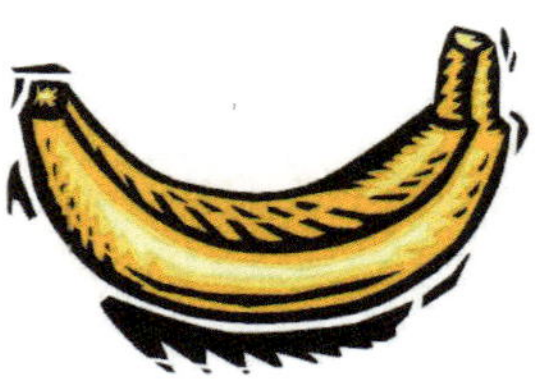

Notice the "speech banana" (the dotted area on the audiogram) and notice how many consonant sounds, such as "f," "t," "th," and "s," are in the higher frequencies. Often one of the first things you become aware of when you start to lose your hearing in the higher frequencies is that people seem to be mumbling. But what's happening is that the consonant sounds become distorted or are not heard at all. Words that have similar sounding consonants are mixed up. Words like tame/came, goat/dote, or share/chair can sound the same. Consonants give speech its clarity and meaning, so when they become jumbled up, it can be frustrating to try to follow a conversation. Vowels can be tricky too–you could even mistake "boot" for "beet"! That's because the pitches that make the vowels in those words sound different may be out of your hearing range.

Don't be discouraged if you find all of this to be as clear as mud!

Gallaudet University* conducted a survey of audiology patients a few years ago and discovered that by the time patients had left the audiologist's office they had forgotten 50 percent of what they were told about their hearing loss, and by the time they got home they had forgotten all of it* (except, of course, the cost of the hearing aids!). ***It's advisable to have someone go with you who can take notes for you to review later.***

**Numerous studies in other areas of medical, legal and financial information also support this finding.*

Audiogram

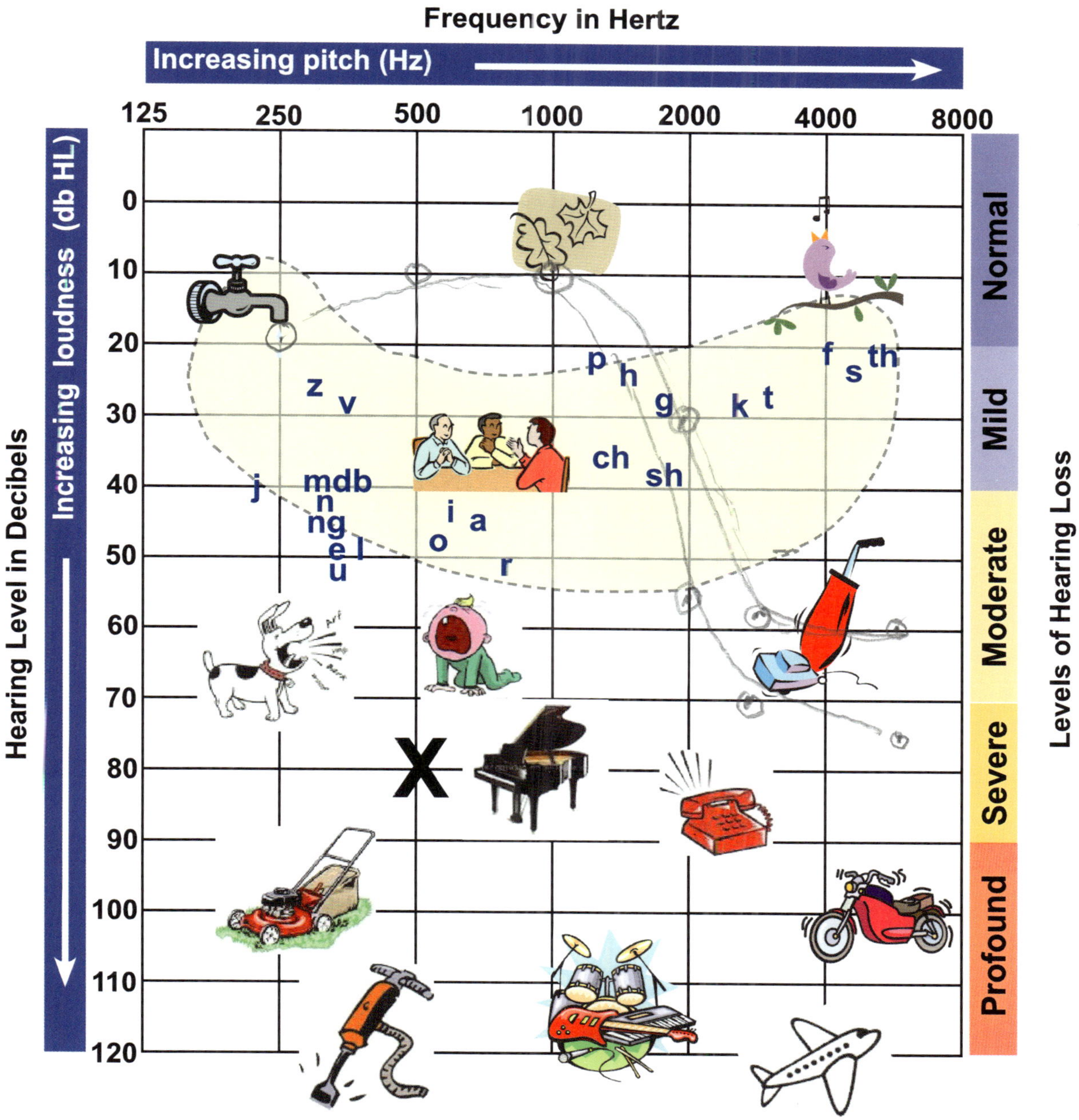

Frequency in Hertz
Increasing pitch (Hz)
125
250
500
1000
2000
4000
8000
Hearing Level in Decibels
Increasing loudness (db HL)
0
10
20
30
40
50
60
70
80
90
100
110
120
Levels of Hearing Loss
Normal
Mild
Moderate
Severe
Profound
z v
p h
g
k t
f s th
ch
sh
j
mdb
n
ng
e l
u
i a
o
r
X

OK, I Need Hearing Aids. . .

What are my choices and how much are they?

There are four **styles** of hearing aids (style refers to their size and what they look like).

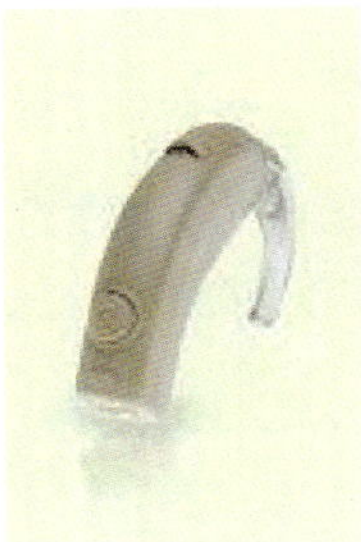

Behind The Ear (BTE). This self-contained unit sits behind the ear with a little tube connected to the ear mold. This style is good for all levels of hearing loss and can accommodate all circuits and options available. Variations of this, which work better for milder losses, include:

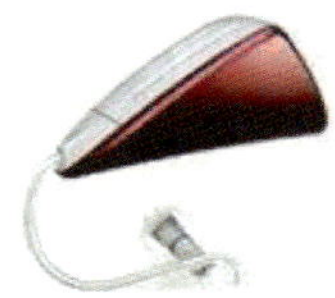

Receiver In the Canal (RIT)

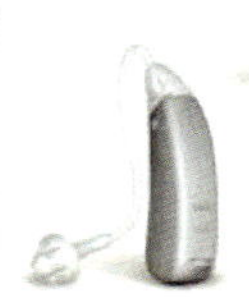

Open fit or slim tube

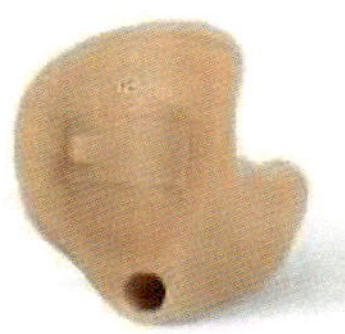

In The Ear (ITE). This self-contained unit fills the entire bowl area of the ear and is used for all levels of hearing loss. It's easy to insert and remove and can accommodate all available circuits and options. This is the most adjustable and strongest of models that fit in the ear.

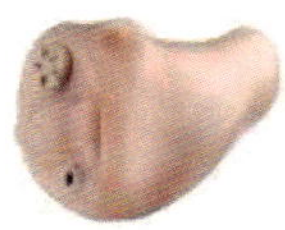

In The Canal (ITC). This self-contained unit fills the outer portion of the ear canal and sits within the bowl area, filling only half of it. This style is used for mild to moderate losses and can be awkward to handle due to its small size. Volume control is often available for this style but not the telecoil (details are on page 17).

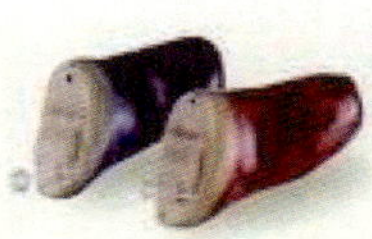

Completely in the Canal (CIC). This is the smallest hearing aid available; it fits deep into the ear canal with a little filament handle for easy removal. This works best for mild to moderate losses but can be difficult to handle due to its very small size. This style cannot accommodate a telecoil.

The Cros and Bi-Cros hearing aid comes in BTE and ITE styles. It transmits sound from a microphone near one ear to a receiver on the other ear and is recommended when there is no useful hearing in one ear.

It is often very tempting to assign more importance to what the hearing aids LOOK like than to what they will accomplish. Audiologists observe that "clients buy their first hearing aids for cosmetic reasons, but the second pair of hearing aids they buy to hear with."

There are three **types** of hearing aids (type refers to the circuitry and technology).

Conventional Analog. This is the old war horse of hearing aids; it simply amplifies the sounds you hear, and the professional can adjust the sound to your comfort level with a tiny screwdriver setting. The current cost of an analog aid is typically $700 to $1,100.

Digitally Programmable Analog. The sound is still amplified through an analog circuit, but there is usually greater control over the adjustments to match your hearing loss. Some have more than one listening program. By pressing a button on the aid, you can cause the aid to amplify in a different way for a noisy room, on the phone, for music or when in a quiet room. Current prices for this type of hearing aid are typically between $1,000 and $2,000.

Fully digital. Sound picked up by this hearing aid is amplified on a computer chip inside the aid. The result is usually a cleaner, sharper speech sound with the greatest control over the adjustments that can be made and the separation of desired speech from undesirable noise. A fully digital hearing aid currently costs between $1,100 and $3,500.

I've decided to get hearing aids. Now what?

Now comes the most important part of this whole hearing aid adventure. This is what **should** happen.

Once your hearing has been assessed, your professional will use the results of your hearing test to educate you about your hearing loss and explain in simple terms why you have been having difficulty hearing in certain listening situations. The two of you will work together to establish a set of realistic objectives and expectations for improved hearing based on how much hearing loss you have, how long you have had it, and how much help you can reasonably expect from hearing aids.

Your professional will then recommend the type and style of hearing aids that should work best for you, and create the program settings for your hearing aids on his or her computer. How well you adjust to your hearing aids will be dependent on (1) your understanding of your own hearing loss, (2) your realistic expectations for improved hearing with the hearing aids, (3) the hearing aid programming expertise of your professional, and (4) consistent use of your hearing aids.

Hearing aids are an investment. What do I need to know?

You should expect to be sold hearing aids that are new and in good working order, comfortable, and properly adjusted to your hearing loss during your trial period. Under Federal law, you get 30 days to try new hearing aids.

You will sign a sales contract that will have the information about the hearing aids, such as the serial number, manufacturer, sales price, and details of non-refundable costs if you return the hearing aids within the trial period.

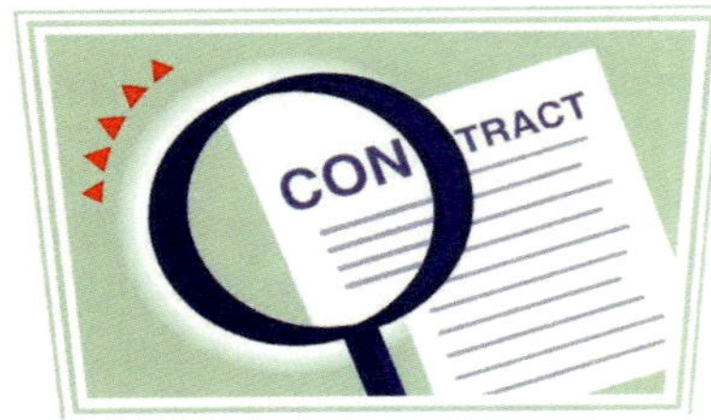

You should also receive written information about terms of payment, service warranty or insurance options for the hearing aid, the full name and address of the hearing professional, and his or her state hearing aid dispenser's license number. Information about hearing aid repairs and how to care for your hearing aids should also be included, as well as an owner's manual.

As you adjust to your new hearing aids, you can expect to return to your professional at least twice during the adjustment period to refine their performance. It helps to keep a journal of your hearing in different places or with different voices. You'll discuss this with your audiologist at the recheck appointments. Based on what you report, he or she will adjust the aids. After your adjustment period is over, you should see your audiologist about every 6 months to clean and check the hearing aids. This keeps them working well and gives you the opportunity to have adjustments made as necessary.

It is important to realize that there is no such thing as "best" hearing aids because our hearing losses are as unique and individual as our fingerprints. What works well for one hearing aid wearer might not work as well for someone else. It is also important to understand that wearing hearing aids will not restore your hearing to normal the way eyeglasses restore sight, and will not prevent further hearing loss.

One or two hearing aids?

If you have hearing loss in both ears, wearing two hearing aids helps with locating where sounds are coming from and provides a stereo effect as you listen to sounds around you. The sound is fuller and richer. Your audiologist can help you make the best decision for your personal situation.

Wait! Can't I buy cheap hearing aids through the mail?

Some people with extremely mild hearing losses have been known to benefit from "mail order" hearing devices. But the devices are often uncomfortable because they are not custom made for your ears. Also, if you haven't had your hearing professionally evaluated, you have no way to know if your hearing problem can be treated medically or if that type of hearing device will work for your type of hearing loss.

How about batteries?

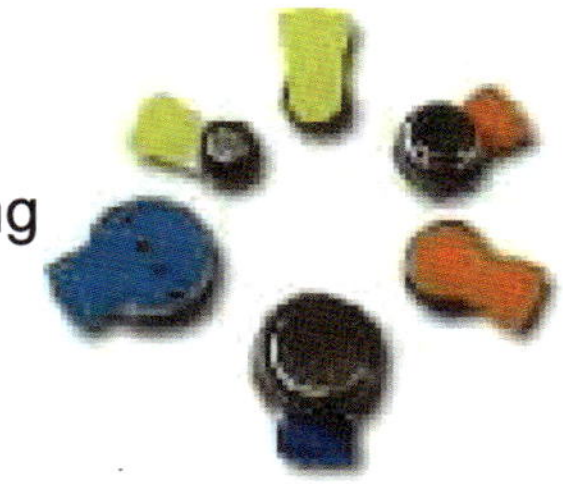

Hearing aid batteries are critical to the functioning of your hearing aid. Batteries will typically last from 5 to 14 days, depending on their size.

Batteries come in four sizes, with corresponding colors and numbers to help you identify them.

Yellow Tab	Size 10	Orange Tab	Size 13
Brown Tab	Size 312	Blue Tab	Size 675

Remember that the **smaller** the battery, the **shorter** the life of the battery.

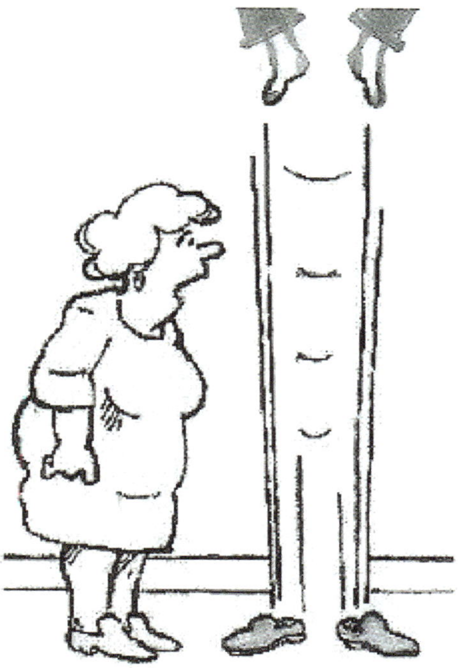

"DID YOU REMEMBER TO GET A NEW BATTERY FOR YOUR HEARING AID?"

Don't leave home without them!

Hearing aids depend on battery power, and sometimes fail at the most inconvenient time. Carry a spare battery with you and change batteries before going to a special event.

Troubleshooting

Sometimes moisture or oil can collect on the surface of the battery so it can't make good contact. Or sometimes the adhesive from the sticker stays stuck on the battery. You may wipe it off with a DRY tissue or cloth to remove residue. If the battery contacts inside the hearing aid have oils on them, have your hearing aid dispenser clean them professionally. This can usually be done in the office.

Aren't you glad modern hearing aids don't use gigantic batteries like this 1.2 pound monster that was used in carbon hearing aids in the 1920s? At the same time, don't miss the tiny modern hearing aid battery near the bottom right corner of the big one. What a contrast! Picture courtesy www.hearingaidmuseum.com.

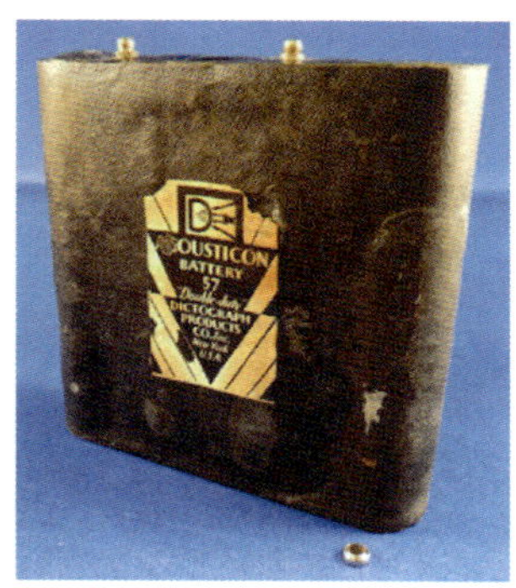

You mentioned a telecoil? What's that?

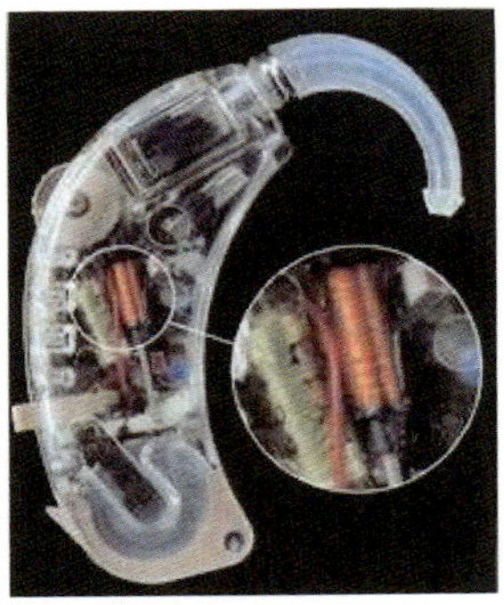

The telecoil is a tiny electromagnet inside the hearing aid. It reacts with external electromagnetic fields such as the signal on a telephone or an induction loop used in large meeting rooms or in public places where assistive listening systems are installed, such as houses of worship, libraries, museums, etc. (more about loops on page 23).

A number of personal assistive listening devices can be used with a telecoil to add a highly desirable dimension to wearing a hearing aid. All you have to do is push a button on your hearing aid to activate it. Some telecoils activate automatically.

A telecoil is also called a T-switch or telephone switch. You should discuss with your professional if a telecoil could benefit your hearing loss. Sometimes audiologists overlook discussing this feature with their patients, and it's important that you know about this valuable option.

How do I get used to my new hearing aids? They're driving me crazy!

Well, let's think about what's happening to your auditory system and it will all make sense. The area of your brain which controls your hearing *(auditory cortex)* has been sort of snoozing for a while because your inner ear and/or auditory nerve hasn't been able to send the sound signals to your brain. Consequently, you've been missing a lot of every day sounds, possibly for years. When you start wearing hearing aids, all of a sudden there are long-forgotten sounds being transmitted to your brain, waking it up from its snooze and taking it by surprise. "Wow!" your brain says, "I haven't heard that for a long time!" Some of this experience can be fun and exciting for you, hearing sounds you haven't heard for ages, but if you start to feel bombarded by all the newness, it's okay to take a break for an hour or so, and try again later.

The good news here is that the auditory cortex is flexible and can adjust to amplification, even after years of silence. It is useful to note that the longer the silence, the longer it may take for the brain to adjust. But with perseverance, results can be encouraging.

You Have to Wear Them!

People who wear their hearing aids consistently during their 30- or 60-day trial period have the most success adjusting to them. Getting used to your hearing aids requires wearing them, wearing them, wearing them, from the time you get up in the morning until you go to bed at night. Not just for book club, not just for bridge or dinner with a friend, but all the time. Eventually you will notice that you don't even realize your hearing aids are in; sounds will start to become more normalized because your brain will have figured out how to handle all this new information and interpret the sounds for you in ways that you can more easily identify.

It is also important to understand what happens when you **do** get used to your new hearing aids. Some people find that after a few months, they don't think their hearing aids are "working as well" as they did in the beginning. A good analogy for this is to think of sitting for hours in a room that's dark—pitch black. Then someone turns on a low light and that seems more than adequate because you've been used to sitting in the dark. But when your eyes adjust to that low level of light, it won't be quite enough to read by, so you need the light turned up more. And when you adjust to **that** level, you'll need the light to be even brighter, and so on, until you have a normal level of light. With hearing aids, your brain becomes trained to recognize sounds at a certain level of amplification, and you become smarter about what you're listening to. The hearing aids haven't changed; you have! And that's good news! Eventually you just need to have your hearing aid amplification adjusted to a new level.

Caring for your hearing aids

- Always keep them dry
- When not in use, **store in a container**, away from heat, moisture and the family pet
- Remove the battery or open the battery door when you take your hearing aid out; this extends the life of the battery
- Clean your hearing aid every day with cleansing wipes available from your audiologist
- Use a tiny loop tool to remove wax from the in-the-ear aid or change your wax guard as instructed by your audiologist
- Do not drop your hearing aid on a hard surface; it could crack the shell and damage the circuits
- If you wear BTE aids, inspect the tube for cracks or moisture build-up. Use a loop tool to remove wax from the tube. Have your tubing replaced by your audiologist every 6-9 months

Bert: I got this great new hearing aid the other day.

Chad: Are you wearing it now?

Bert: Yup. Cost me $4,000, but it's top of the line.

Chad: What kind is it?

Bert: 12:30.

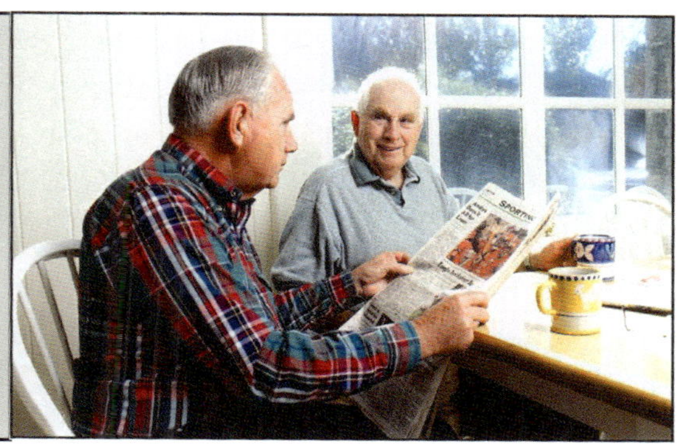

The Ongoing Quest for my "Perfect" Hearing Aid

By Lenore Benderly, Longboat Key, Florida

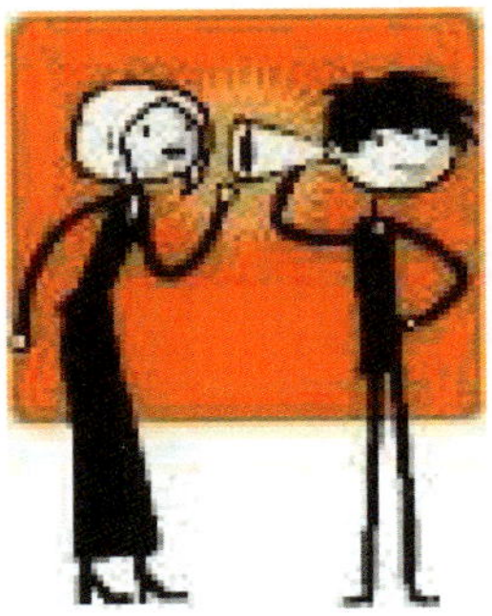

About four years ago, I was seated at a table for eight women from many parts of the world at a Unifem luncheon. Suddenly, I could not hear what the woman on my left was saying to me. At that moment I lost all the hearing in my left ear due to an acoustic neuroma which had grown on my acoustic and vestibular nerves. I rushed to see an ENT who told me that single-sided deafness was a common occurrence in acoustic neuroma cases, and there was nothing to do to recover my hearing in the left ear. The loss of balance was recoverable because my brain could be retrained to take over that job from the non-functioning left vestibular nerve. After I had gamma knife surgery to treat the neuroma, I worked hard at physical therapy and eventually recovered my balance totally. I am happy to report that I can play tennis and have had no further falls from loss of balance. And the acoustic neuroma has not grown any larger.

Since the hearing in my right ear was normal, I was able to function fairly well for a couple of years—I just did not know where the sound was coming from, who was talking to me, where the horn was honking, etc. I could only hear sweet nothings and secrets in the right ear.

Then the hearing in my right ear began to decline, probably due to aging. Now I was missing punch lines, not enjoying movies and TV, having difficulty understanding friends if there were more than two or three in the group. I was feeling more and more isolated. I visited the audiologist whose office was part of my ENT's domain with a request for a hearing aid for my "good" ear. During these two years, I tried and returned at least six hearing aids in the quest to find hearing improvement, comfort and simplicity of use.

Amy, my audiologist, continues to be very patient and accommodating. She understands how personal and difficult it can be to find a good choice. I have visited her every week or every other week for two years. Several times, I thought I had found the right hearing aid but it turned out to have some deficiency. The only way to find a good fit is to keep trying.

Go back to your audiologist and have the hearing aid retested and readjusted until you are certain you are satisfied. I even gave up and took several months off because I was so disappointed with all the results. I told Amy to let me know when some new technology came forth that might improve my chances. And she did. The products are changing all the time and they are improving. I finally am wearing a hearing aid that is comfortable, simple to operate, and quite clear with normal sounds. I have succeeded in my quest for a satisfactory right side hearing aid at last.

As for my left side, I am happy to report that after several unsuccessful attempts, I now seem to have found a hearing aid for that ear which is helping me to hear better. Amy, my audiologist, is very pleased and quite surprised. My advice is: find a competent and patient audiologist and persevere even if it takes years! It is certainly worth the effort.

Assistive Listening Devices to the Rescue

Understanding assistive listening devices means learning about (1) what they do and (2) how they work. Lise Hamlin shared her story with us about the different listening devices she has used over the years. We invited Dr. Neil Bauman, who has written extensively about hearing assistive technology, to introduce and amplify segments of Lise's story by describing how these devices work.

Dr. Neil says . . .

Hearing aids can improve your ability to participate in many listening situations, but they are not perfect. They are not designed to overcome the problems we face when we are some distance from the person speaking or when we are in a noisy place such as a busy restaurant. That's where Assistive Listening Devices (ALDs) come in. They offer two major benefits. First, they can help cut out the surrounding noise and bring the sounds closer to you so you can hear and understand a lot better. You hear more of the high-frequency consonant sounds that give speech its meaning. This makes a huge difference to your understanding people talking. Second, ALDs can be used with or without your hearing aids!

Let's join *Lise Hamlin* as she describes her personal journey with ALDs.

My First Assistive Listening Devices

By Lise Hamlin

I lost my hearing literally overnight about 25 years ago. When that happened, I didn't know the first thing about how to function as a person with a significant hearing loss in a hearing world. I think most people who age into their hearing loss feel the same way: they know what it's like to be able to hear, but they don't know what they need to know to have a full life after a hearing loss. It can be done. It takes time and patience, but it can be done.

Portable Telephone Amplifier

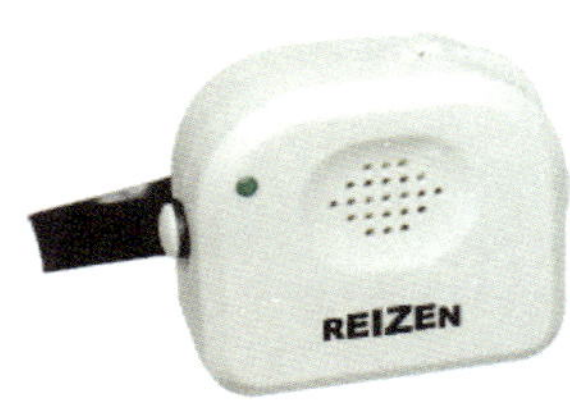

The first thing I wanted was help hearing on the phone, so I bought a portable amplifier. It was a small AT&T amplifier that looked similar to the one pictured here:

That was a great help when I traveled and needed to make a call to someone from my hotel room or from a public phone (well, that was then—try to find a public phone now!) It was small, worked with AA or AAA batteries, and it was easy to use. It was great. I could pop that into my suitcase and I was good to go. These portable amplifiers now sell for between $20 and $30.

I learned later that there is another amplifier, an "in-line" amplifier, that not only has a volume control that allows you to increase the volume quite a bit, but also has a tone control. That means if someone speaks in a pitch I can't hear very well, I can change the tone right on the amplifier. It works on a 9 volt battery and costs about $35. The great thing is that it's portable and works with any corded phone.

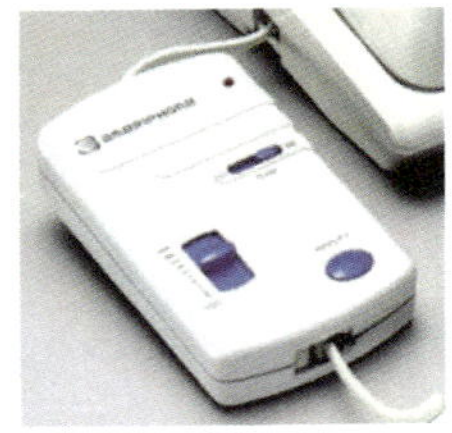

Amplified Telephones

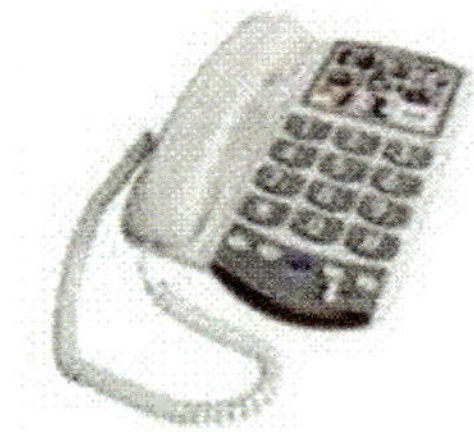

The portable amplifier was great, but not what I wanted to use at home. At home I wanted to be able to pick up the phone as soon as it rang—I didn't want to have to strap on the amplifier every time I needed it. And I wanted to see if there was a phone that was even better than the in-line amplifier. So I had to look around some more. What I found next was an amplified phone with large buttons.

The new phone I got not only had a volume control for the handset and large dial pad so I could see the numbers and letters easily, but also had a loud ringer, which was another big help. Today, there are also cordless phones with caller ID and a range of helpful features like an answering machine in the phone itself.

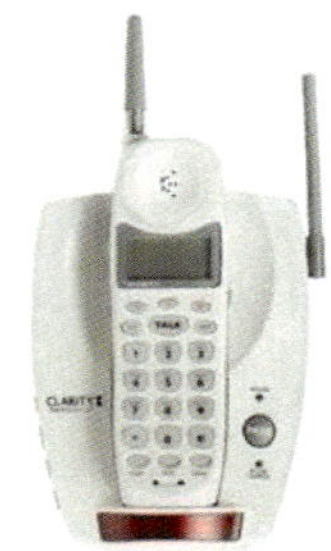

Captioned Telephones

Now I use CapTel and Web CapTel phone systems. The CapTel phone looks and works like a regular phone, but also has a window display to read the conversation.

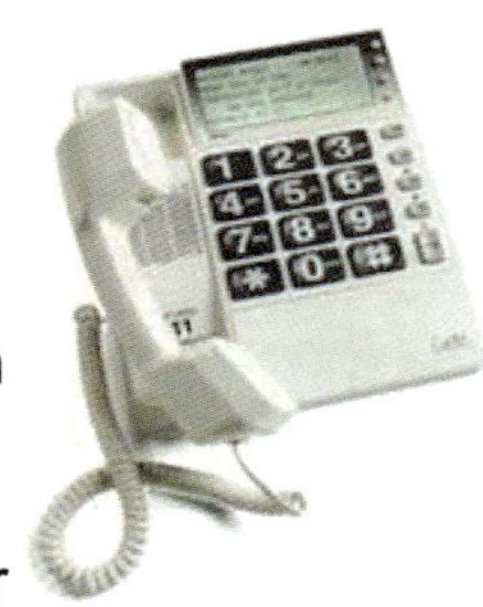

A specially trained operator at the CapTel captioning service puts your call through and then transcribes everything the other party says into written text, using the latest in voice-recognition technology. The written text appears on a bright, easy-to-read display window built into the CapTel phone. The captions appear almost simultaneously with the spoken word, allowing you to understand everything that is said—either by hearing it or by reading it, or both. At no time are you aware of someone else on the line; it's completely discreet. The cost of the phone is about $490.

The Web CapTel is offered for **free** by both Sprint and Hamilton Relay. I found it was very simple to use. Just create a "User" account on your computer, log on, and then type in the telephone number you are calling from. The captioner then calls you at that number, and once you are on the line you type in the number of the person you are calling. When the captioner puts you through to your party, you can read what the other person is saying on your computer monitor! You can even adjust the size and color of the font to make it easier to read.

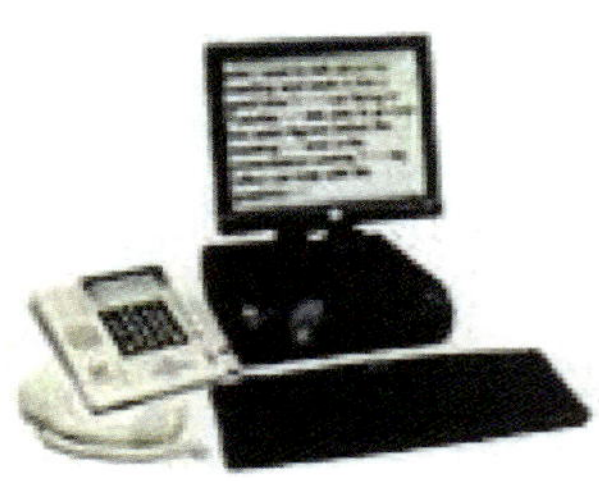

Dr. Neil says . . .

You can also activate your hearing aid t-coils to work with your phone's receiver. This blocks out all background noise on the phone so the voice of the person you are listening to can come in loud and clear. Some special phones have jacks in them so you can plug in a neckloop.

CapTel requires connection to a standard analog telephone line (or analog port), such as is commonly found in households. You cannot connect CapTel to a digital telephone line. The cost of the captioning service is covered by Telecommunications Relay Service (TRS) funds as part of Title IV of the Americans with Disabilities Act (ADA).

Personal Assistive Listening System

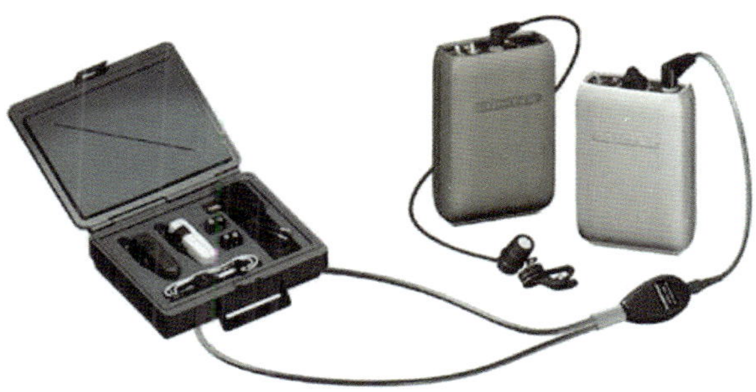

My hearing aid was wonderful, and I was very happy to have it, but it didn't do everything for me in every situation. If I went to a lecture or a meeting, I couldn't hear unless I was in the front row, and the acoustics had to be very good—something that didn't seem to happen very often. If I went out to dinner with a small group of friends, all I could hear was the background noise, and forget about large family dinners! I could barely hear the person sitting next to me. So, I decided I needed some more help.

What I found was a personal FM system. The person speaking needs to wear a small microphone clipped to his or her shirt or blouse. The microphone is attached to a small transmitter. The transmitter sends the sound to a receiver I hold. The receiver sends the sound to my neckloop or headset. I can control the volume of the sound on my receiver and on my hearing aid, so I get the boost I need. And the microphone doesn't pick up all the sound around like my hearing aid does: it just picks up the sound closest to the microphone.

Now I can go to a noisy restaurant with a friend or a meeting or even to church: as long as the person speaking is willing to wear that mike and the transmitter that it's connected to, I can get the sound I need by using the receiver and linking it to my neck loop. Then I turn my hearing aid to the telecoil switch and I can hear everything. It's been great. And the system I bought 25 years ago is still working today! I have had to replace the microphone once and the neckloop twice, but the expensive parts are the same.

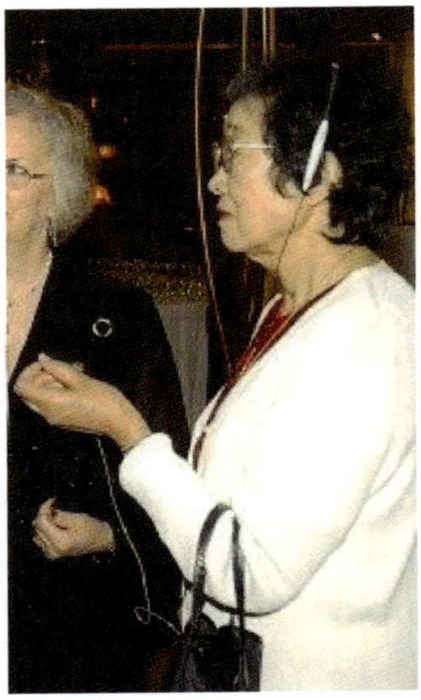

Dr. Neil says . . .

FM systems use radio waves to transmit the sound from the speaker's mouth to your ears. Because there are no wires connecting you to the speaker, you are free to move around, or sit at some distance from the speaker. For example, you can typically be up to 150 feet away from the speaker and still hear just as well as if the person was talking directly into your ears. If you are in a meeting and the people around you are coughing, talking, clinking dishes or rustling papers, your hearing aids will pick this up, and you will have trouble understanding the speaker though all this extraneous noise. With an FM system, you will only hear the sounds going into the speaker's microphone, not the disturbing noise around you.

You can use FM systems even if you have to go into an adjacent room, or if you are outside walking, or riding your bicycle with a friend. One drawback of FM systems is that they tend to be quite expensive—in the neighborhood of $800 and up.

What's a neckloop? A neckloop takes the place of a headset if you have a telecoil on your hearing aid. It's literally a loop of wire that plugs into the receiver, then goes around your neck, like a necklace (but, for you guys, it doesn't look like a necklace — it looks like a wire!). When you turn on the receiver and turn on your telecoil switch, the sound gets sent over the wire and is picked up by the telecoil in your hearing aid. It works very well!

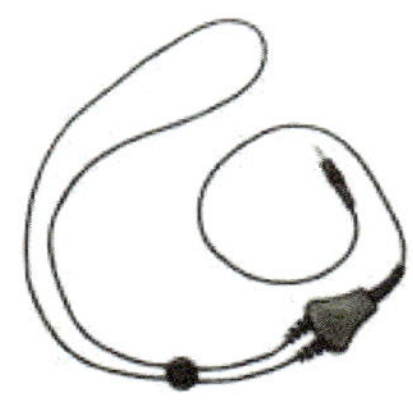

Dr. Neil says . . .

Induction loops "connect" to your hearing aids via the t-coils—there is no physical connection. You can plug a neckloop into whatever device you are listening to—whether a personal amplifier or an FM or infrared receiver, or directly into a radio or MP3 player or iPod.

There are also "room loops." The typical application for room loops is for meetings and for listening to the TV. If you install a room loop in your house, you can freely move around anywhere inside the loop and still hear the TV as if you are right in front of it, as long as you have your hearing aid t-coil activated. Room loops are relatively inexpensive—under $200.

Look for this symbol to alert you if a room is looped and you can use your t-coil. It is usually located at the entrance to the room.

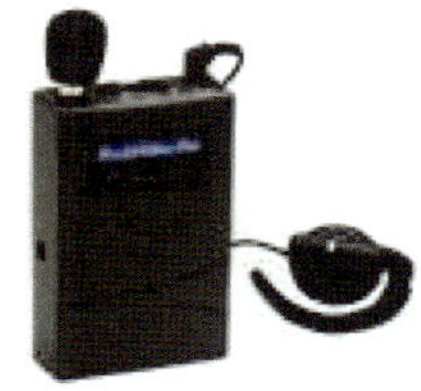

Now, some people may not need the power the FM system gives me; they may do fine with a smaller version like a "PockeTalker." The advantage of this smaller unit is that it is much less expensive. But there are disadvantages. It doesn't have a transmitter and a receiver; it doesn't send the signal anywhere, it depends on wires to get the sound from the microphone to the headset or neckloop. That means you must be close to the person speaking, within wireline distance.

You can use it in a restaurant, but you can't put it on the lectern where a lecture is given—the wires aren't that long! It also seems to be better for people who have a mild or perhaps a moderate hearing loss, but it generally doesn't work well for a severe to profound hearing loss.

Dr. Neil says . . .

You clip a lapel microphone to the person to whom you are conversing, plug it into your personal amplifier, plug in a neckloop and listen to your partner via the t-coils in your hearing aids. This cuts out most of the background noise.

The downside of such an arrangement is that you are wired together and thus are not free to move around. You can also use these devices to listen to your TV by attaching the microphone of the device near the TV's speaker and running the microphone cord across the room to your personal amplifier. You can do the same if the person you are talking to is sitting on the other side of the room. This is typically the cheapest way to go. Cost is around $200 with the lapel microphone.

Television

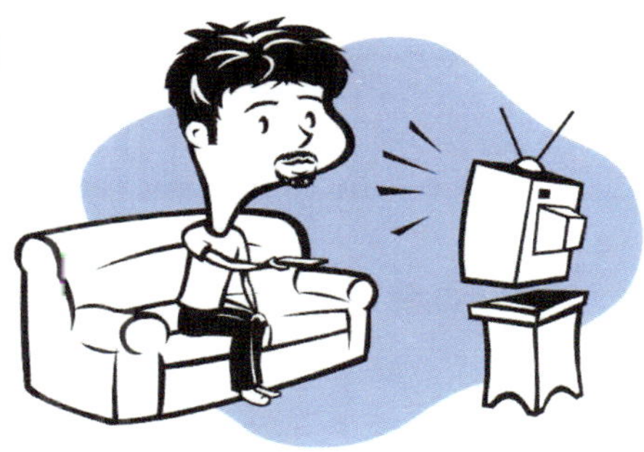

Now that I had what I needed to help me understand on the phone and be able to talk to my friends one to one and go to meetings, the next thing I wanted in my life was to be reconnected to the rest of the world. I wanted my television back. I wanted to hear the news and the weather report, and I wanted to be able to relax with my family watching television shows—and know why they were all laughing.

The first thing I did was to get a television that has closed captioning. All televisions manufactured in the U.S. with a screen 13 inches or larger are required to have closed captioning. What is not required is a closed captioning button right on your remote. So you might have to search for the captioning in the menu of your television setup, but if the TV is large enough, the captioning just needs to be found.

That was all great, but there were times when other people would be watching TV with me who didn't really like reading the captions. I realized I could use my FM system by simply putting the microphone close to the television's loudspeaker. That wasn't bad, but I found that there are systems that are designed specifically for being able to listen to the television. Twenty-five years ago, I knew of only one system. There are several systems available now. To name just a few:

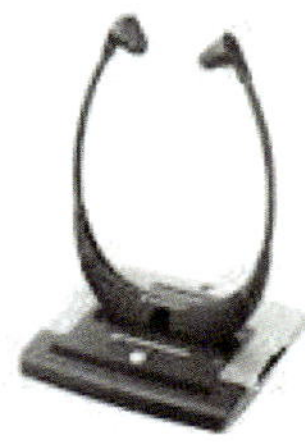

- Clarity C120 Wireless TV Amplifier CL-C120
- ClearSounds CS2000M UltraClear TV Listening System HT-CS2000M
- Sennheiser IS 410 Infrared Stereo TV System HC-IS410
- TV EARS Pro Headset System TVEARS-PRO

These range in price from $70 to $200. A few of these simply send the TV's sound to your ears, others have fancier features. But, they all run on Infrared (IR) light, just like your remote control runs on IR light. They are easy to set up and most people find the sound very good. They offer another way to hear TV, without having to read the captions, or turn up the volume so loud everyone else is blasted out of the room.

Those were among the first devices I got to help me hear. I was able to hear better, able to hold down a job, even get a new job when the time came. And I could still watch my favorite television shows. As I say, I love my hearing aid, but I also love all the new technology!

Dr. Neil says . . .

Infrared systems are similar to FM systems, except they use light waves instead of radio waves to transmit the sound. Typically, infrared receivers are used in meeting halls/theaters and for watching TV.

However, infrared systems are not as versatile as FM systems because of two things. First, you cannot use them outside or in a room with a lot of sunlight streaming in—as the infrared component of the sun's rays causes horrible interference. So do many flat-screen TVs. Second, light waves travel in straight lines. Thus your infrared receiver always has to be line-of-sight to the speaker's infrared transmitter (called an emitter). Therefore, if you turn away from the TV, or go to the kitchen, you won't hear anything until you return and face the TV. Anything or anybody coming between you and the emitter blocks the signal.

Assistive Listening Devices have been one of the best kept secrets in town—but no longer!

Now that you know how useful they can be, avail yourself of their benefits. When used with your hearing aids in difficult listening situations, the two make an awesome combination!

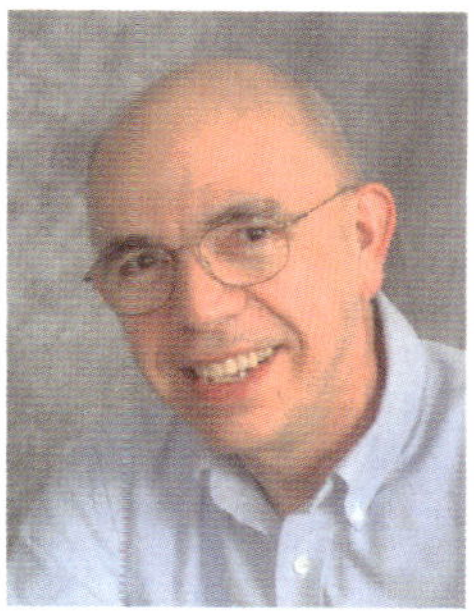

Neil G. Bauman, Ph.D. (Dr. Neil) *directs The Center for Hearing Loss Help www.hearinglosshelp.com in Stewartstown, PA. Neil has successfully lived with a severe hearing loss all his life. The Center helps people also live successful and fulfilling lives in spite of their hearing losses by providing them with information, counsel, quality books and carefully selected assistive devices that help them successfully deal with hearing loss and other ear-related problems.*

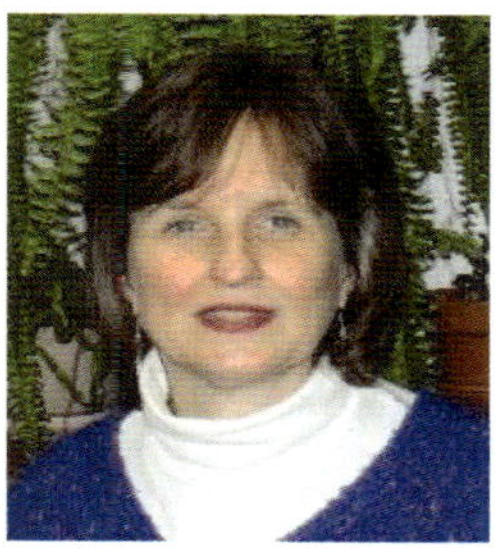

Lise Hamlin *joined the Hearing Loss Association of America's national staff as Director of Public Policy and State Development in April, 2008. She has a strong background in advocacy and working with people with disabilities having been with the League for the Hard of Hearing in New York City and most recently with NVRC where she served as the Director of Access & Advocacy and was an instructor for TDI's emergency preparedness course.*

Did you know?...

Title III of the **Americans with Disabilities Act (ADA)** gives rights of equal access to places of public accommodation for people who are deaf and hard of hearing. This means you have the right to receive an assistive listening device if you need one!

Be sure to ask for one when you go the movies, the theatre or a museum. Some community-based recreational program planners will require advance notice that you will need a listening system, but don't hesitate to request one. After all, you have the right to enjoy all the same programs that hearing people do!

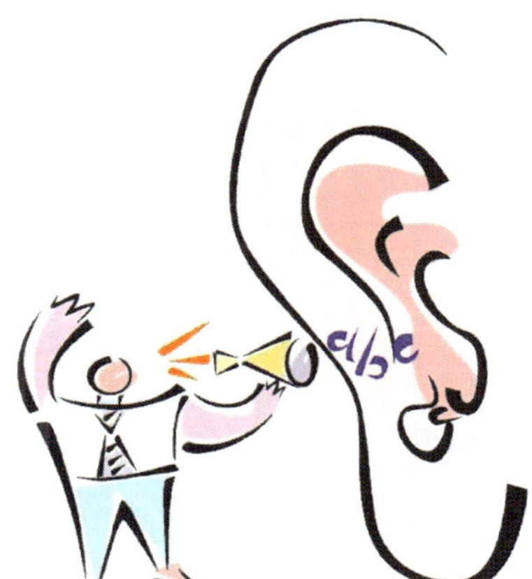

The Silent Screen

By Mike DeFries

I'm an 85 year old man. About 20 years or so ago, I started noticing a strange phenomenon. When seated around a large table, either in a business setting or in a social group such as one at a restaurant, the scene was projected to me in part either as an old silent movie or as a modern talking picture. When certain people held the stage, the screen went silent, while when others were talking the screen sprang to life. At first I would frantically scramble to follow everything that was said with "what, what?" More recently I became reconciled to missing major portions of the conversation while nodding sagaciously from time to time. Occasionally I would blurt out a non-sequitur, but these usually passed in the flow of conversation.

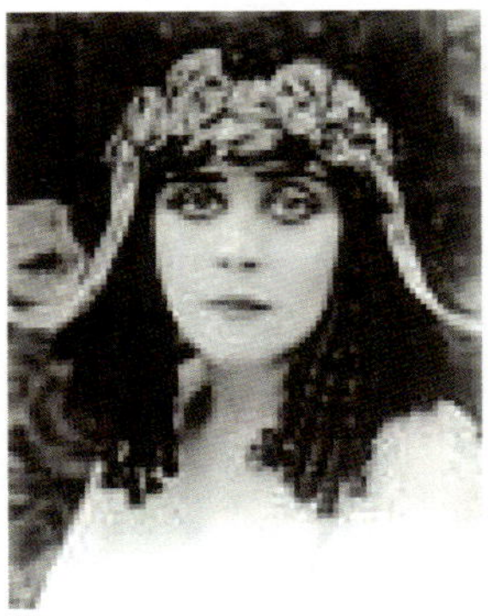

Not my mother! Really!

There seems to be a definite line between those who star in the talking version, and those who invoke the silent movie era. At the present state of my hearing, perhaps half of the people I interact with have become Theda Baras. Oddly, when the scene reverts to the silent movies, the body language of the actors seems to mimic the exaggerations of the actors of the bygone era.

One cannot always predict who will perform as a "low" talker. There doesn't seem to be a gradation between the two. Someone is in one category or another; either I get it or I don't. Generally, but not exclusively, more women than men are in the "low talker" category. It is difficult to predict which individuals will fall into one category or the other from one-to-one conversations compared to a group setting.

Pocket Talkers have been recommended to me to overcome the "large table" situation. I've tried them several times, and by and large they do provide the advertised amplification of the sound. They only cost about $200. Why then haven't I bought one? Let me try to explain — I don't really know. The money is certainly not the reason. Then it must be something else. One reason I cite to myself is that I do not really want to draw attention to my infirmity. The other is that hearing devices inevitably distort the received sound, usually in unpleasant ways. A third reason is that I am just a stubborn guy; I'm not willing to succumb to the inevitable yet.

If I am stubborn, I inherited it from my mother. For the last 25 years of her life, my mother suffered increasing hearing loss. During the last ten or so, her hearing loss became almost total. She also suffered severely from tinnitus. (I do too, but fortunately for me it is only a nuisance, at least in my present stage of hearing loss.) My mother passed away at the age of 95, firmly convinced that all TV manufacturers entered into a conspiracy to damage the audio of her set just to torment her.

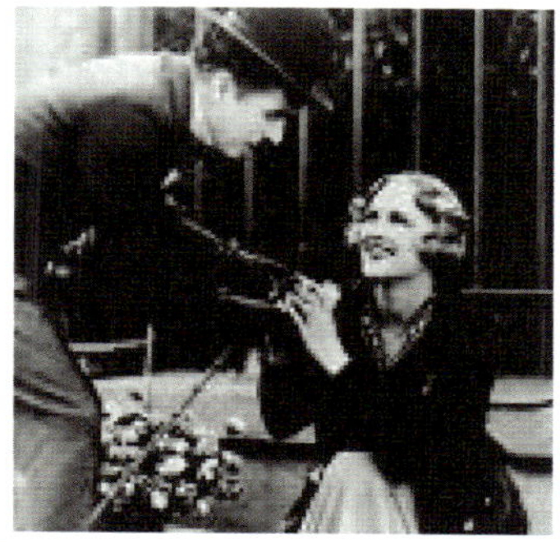

When silence was golden

At some point, she somewhat secretly consented to be fitted with a hearing aid, but only so she could participate in the daily convocation of her cronies on their favorite park bench. But gradually this group evaporated from frailty or death.

My mother's only hope of communicating with the world at-large became, somehow, coaxing understandable communication from the "non-existent' sound system of her TV. At this point, concentrating on lip reading from the TV images or from the sketchy captions available at the time became her only hope, but even this was often interrupted by extremely loud screeching sounds from her so-called hearing aid of that day. But she never gave up hope that someday things would return to normal.

One thing I learned from my mother was how stress could play an important role in hearing loss. She had been brought to a clinic for a check-up. The doctor she expected to see was not there, bringing on complete loss of hearing and an unusual complete loss of the ability to communicate with her. The situation was only resolved by another very experienced doctor familiar with this condition.

While I see my mother's constant battle with hearing loss as courageous, my own reaction to hearing loss is largely stubborn. But not completely so; I have the loudest door bell chime that Home Depot has to offer, and it works for me. I have found an AT&T wireless speaker phone that is loud enough for me and possibly the entire neighborhood. But best of all, I have installed a pair of Bose speakers ($70 for the pair at BJ's) to replace my puny TV audio system. I am sure that with increasing years I will have to rely on the wonders of sound amplification to an ever greater and greater extent.

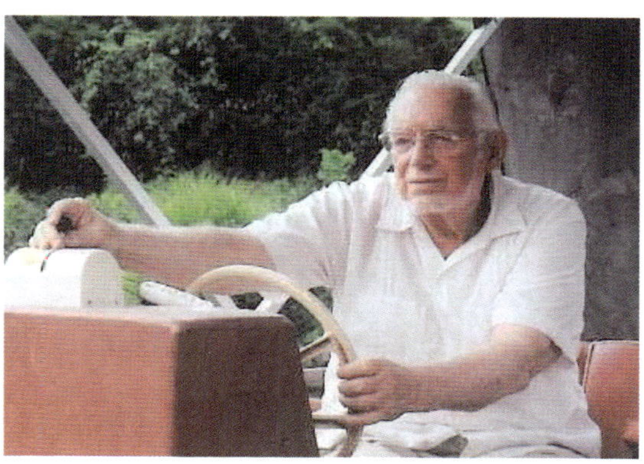

***Mike DeFries** worked on the Manhattan Project as a chemical engineer during World War II. After the war, he came to the Washington, D.C. area to work at the Army Prosthetics Research lab, then at the Walter Reed Annex. He avidly believes that nanotechnology will provide a revolutionary advance to the restoration of hearing in the not too distant future.*

Alerting Devices Can Save Your Life
(and make your life less stressful, too)

By Neil G. Bauman, Ph.D.

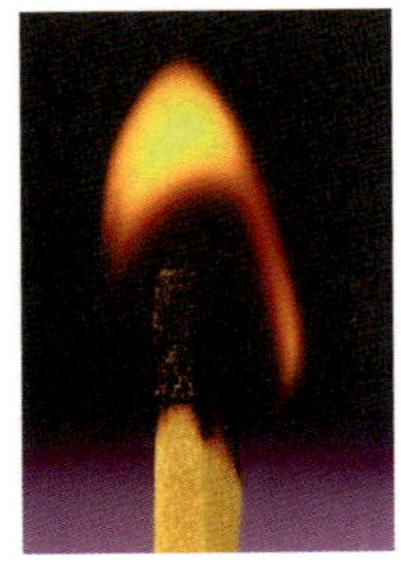

Here in the United States, a house catches fire every 74 seconds!

That's scary!

Even more scary for those of us who have hearing loss is the fact that most fires occur at night when we are sleeping, and our hearing aids and/or cochlear implant headpieces and processors are also peacefully "sleeping" on our bedside tables. Thus, we often cannot hear the smoke detector blaring its warning to us from our bedroom ceilings.

Fire is not the only danger to which we are exposed. Carbon monoxide is an insidious killer that can silently sneak up on us and snuff out our lives while we sleep because again our hearing devices are reposing on the bedside table. Thus, we do not hear our CO detector's shrill warning of impending doom.

During the night a tornado may sweep through our neighborhood, but we may never know it because we can't hear the weather warning blaring from our NOAA weather radios. Instead of immediately taking shelter in our basements, we may become tragic statistics on the next newscast.

Alerting devices aren't only for saving lives. They also make our lives easier. For example, they can alert us to an important phone call when we can't hear the phone ringing, let us know that someone is at the door or even that a sick or bedridden loved one needs our attention.

Because we often can't hear traditional warning alarms, we hard of hearing people need special alerting devices that not only make loud sounds, but also flash lights and vibrate our beds or personal pagers so that even if we miss one or two of the alerting signals, the third one will finally grab our attention so we can take action.

Some alerting devices are "standalone" devices. For example, I have a phone that not only has a loud ringer, but also flashes a light that is plugged into its remote wall module and shakes the bed. I also have a weather alert radio that sounds a loud warning tone and either flashes a light or shakes the bed to awaken me to the fact there might be a tornado barreling down on me while I sleep. You can also get standalone door bells and smoke detectors, etc.

However, if you need a number of these devices, it is much simpler to have a complete integrated system so you only need one bed shaker module and one (or more) flashing lights that will activate whenever any of the alerting devices activates. The best systems even include a vibrating pager you wear on your belt. It will alert you to any of the above warnings, even if you are out in your yard, or in the basement.

Here are some of the "incidents" a good warning system can alert you to:

- fire alarm or smoke detector
- carbon monoxide detector
- weather radio warning (tornado, severe thunderstorm, etc.)
- telephone
- doorbell
- alarm clock
- sound monitor (baby crying, someone calling)
- someone breaking into your house
- sick or bedridden person in your home who needs help now
- warning that someone is leaving their room, especially at night—for example, a loved one with Alzheimer's disease

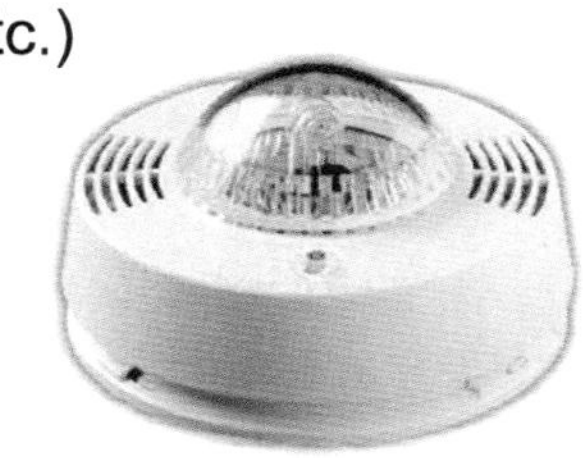

There are a number of alerting systems available, but only the best systems can provide warnings for all of the above situations. Before you buy an alerting system, check that it has the following four characteristics:

- It is reliable. By the same token, you don't want unnecessary false alerts either!

- It has battery backup (in case the emergency occurs when there is a power outage which may well be the case).

- It alerts you in three modes at the same time—sound, light and vibration.

- It is flexible (has all the various alerting modules you need).

If you don't know where to start, I would recommend the Silent Call systems as the most reliable, flexible and attention-getting systems available, starting at about $70.00. You can contact them at Silent Call Communications, 5095 Williams Lake Road, Waterford, Michigan, 48329; 1-800-572-5227.

Note: when you have your alerting system all set up, don't forget that it uses batteries in its various modules, and batteries eventually die. Replace them regularly so your alerting system won't fail just when you really need it.

Technology Assistance Program

By Debbie Jones

The Virginia Department for the Deaf and Hard of Hearing (VDDHH) established the Technology Assistance Program (TAP) to provide assistance to Virginia residents who are deaf, hard of hearing, deafblind, or speech-impaired in getting the telephone equipment they need to stay or become more independent. The TAP program has evolved over the years to meet the changing needs of consumers and fit within the Commonwealth's budget. Its current incarnation is the Loan to Own (L2O) program.

Loan to Own Program (L2O)

For example, let's say that your hearing loss is making it difficult for you to understand speech on a regular telephone. If you can provide proof of Virginia residency, documentation of your hearing loss (usually an audiogram), and if your monthly income meets the L2O guidelines, you could borrow an amplified phone for up to 30 days to see if it works for you. If you are satisfied with the phone after 30 days, it becomes yours.

Devices available through L2O include:

- Text Telephones (TTYs)
- Amplified Telephones
- Voice Carry Over (VCO) Phones
- Captioned Telephones
- Hearing Carry Over (HCO) phones
- Visual Signalers
- Audible Signalers

If you are not eligible for the L2O program, you may still be able to get equipment through TAP at cost. Applications may be obtained through a demonstration site or an Outreach Specialist who can explain the process to you and assist you in filling out the application.

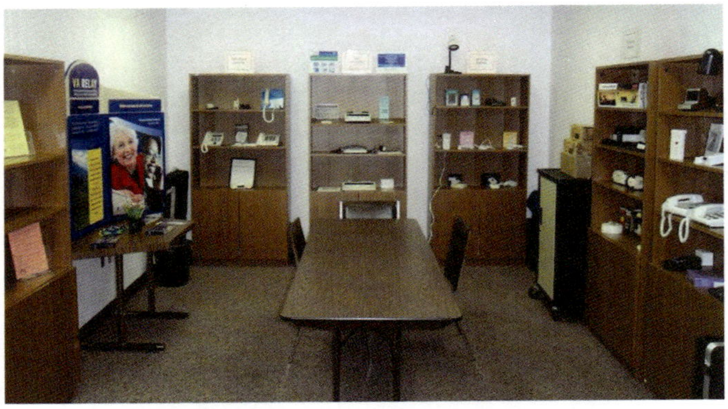

NVRC's Demonstration Room

There is a network of sites across the Commonwealth—like NVRC's demo room—that can demonstrate L2O equipment and help hard of hearing consumers choose the right device for their hearing/listening needs.

NVRC is a demonstration site for the Northern Virginia area which includes Fairfax County, Arlington County, Loudoun County, Prince William County and the Cities of Fairfax, Falls Church, Alexandria, Manassas, and Manassas Park.

For more information about this program or to set up an appointment to determine your eligibility, contact NVRC:

Debbie Jones
Resource/Technology Specialist
703-352-9055, Ext. 101
703-352-9056, TTY
djones@nvrc.org

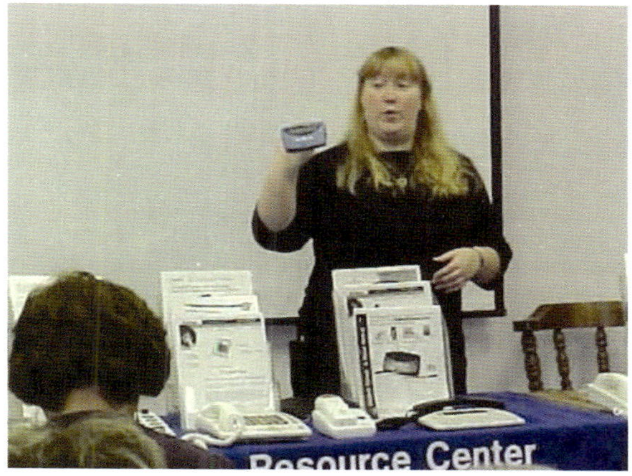

Debbie Jones, *Resource and Technology Specialist. During her 13 years at NVRC, Debbie has given hundreds of technology demonstrations to consumers, administrators, agencies, emergency personnel, educators and students. She studied Psychology at George Washington University, is fluent in American Sign Language, and is the in the testing process to become a nationally certified interpreter.*

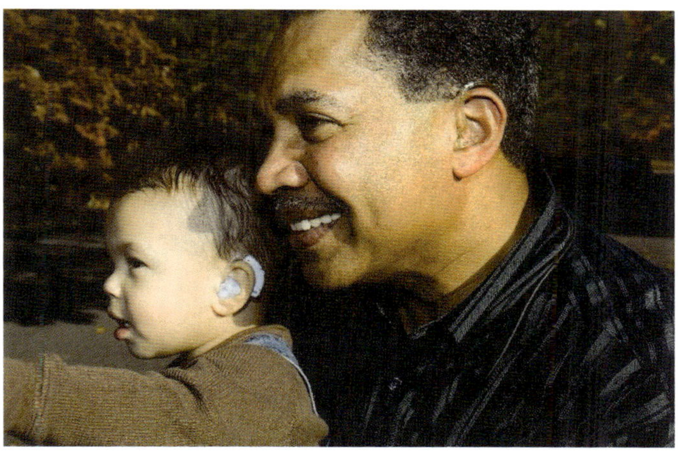

Ron Lanier with his grandson

Virginia Department for Deaf and Hard of Hearing (VDDHH)

1602 Rolling Hills Dr., Suite 203
Richmond, Virginia 23229-5012
(804) 662-9502 V/TTY, Toll Free
(800) 552-7917 V/TTY

Ronald L. Lanier, Director

Virginia Relay DIAL 7-1-1 www.VARelay.org
VDDHH www.vddhh.org
Virginia Relay Partner www.Relaypartner.org

A Cochlear Implant

What is a Cochlear Implant?

A cochlear implant (CI) is an electronic device with three principal elements:

- *A battery-operated external speech processor** that converts sound waves into digital signals
- *A magnetic connector* attached to the side of the head that transmits the signals to the implant
- *An internal implant* surgically placed in the cochlea and linked by a wire to the hearing nerve

*The speech processor is a mini-computer that processes sound waves electronically and sends them to the cochlea so that the sounds can be understood by the brain.

Implants are available in BTE models and body pack versions. Most wearers choose a BTE model.

Who Can Get an Implant?

Candidates for cochlear implants include totally deaf individuals and persons with a severe-to-profound hearing loss who retain some residual speech understanding. Older adults in their 80s and 90s have received CIs, as have infants as young as 12 months.

Qualifying for an Implant

A letter from a physician or audiologist citing "medical necessity" is required to establish implant eligibility. The letter certifies that the patient meets the FDA guidelines of 60 percent or less sentence discrimination in the best aided condition, with 50 percent or less sentence discrimination in the ear being implanted. Medicare requires speech discrimination ability of 40 percent or less in the best aided condition.

Medical Insurance for Implants

As of 2008, cochlear implant surgery can be as high as $70,000. However, many health insurance policies and Medicare underwrite a substantial portion of the implantation costs under "medical necessity" provisions.

Surgical Procedure

The surgery is performed under general anesthesia, usually as an outpatient procedure. The surgeon threads a wire array through the cochlea, where it is linked to the hearing nerve. The wire array transmits the signals in their component speech frequencies. Typically, only one ear is implanted, although dual implants have been installed to meet special needs. The CI will destroy any residual hearing in the implanted ear.

Getting Used to an Implant

Auditory therapy may be required as part of the "breaking in" process, depending on the extent and character of the hearing loss and the recipient's receptivity to the new sounds the implant provides. Some patients find that implants restore improved levels of speech understanding within a day or two without therapy, but others may take weeks or months to reach acceptable levels. Although speech might sound like Donald Duck at first, it soon becomes more "normal."

Implant Manufacturers

The three principal implant manufacturers are:

Cochlear Americas
13059 East Peakview Avenue
Centennial, CO 80111
1-800-523-5798
www.cochlearamericas.com

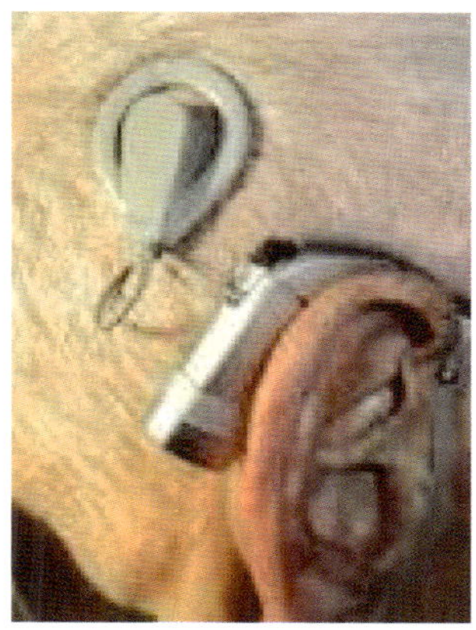

Advanced Bionics
12740 San Fernando Road
Sylmar, CA 91342
1-800-678-2575
www.advancedbionics.com

Med-El Corp. (North America)
25111 Old Cornwallis Road, Suite 100
Durham, NC 27713
1-888-633-3524
www.medel.com

Titanium is the primary product used by the Cochlear Co. for its inserts, while ceramic inserts are used by Advanced Bionics and Med-El.

Thanks to Ben W. Gilbert (deceased), original author and photo, and the Hearing Loss Association of Washington State. Content edited to accommodate space restrictions.

Learning to Hear Again
My Cochlear Implant Adventure

By Joan Cassidy

Let me start by saying that I love my cochlear implant and can't imagine going back to struggling with one deaf ear and the other ear with a hearing aid that only gave me an awareness of sound. So I don't pretend to be objective on the subject. On the other hand, getting an implant is no walk in the park. You don't just have the surgery and turn on the processor and hear like you did when you were 25. Come to think of it, when I was that age I already had a mild to moderate hearing loss so in my case it's probably true that I now hear like when I was 25.

It took me a couple of years to make the decision. I went to a lot of workshops and talked to people with CIs. The thought of surgery on my head was not appealing but after watching a video of an actual CI surgery and talking to Dr Niparko from the Johns Hopkins Listening Center, I was reassured that this was not "brain surgery." The internal part of the implant would be under the skin behind my ear with a thin filament going into my inner ear.

I think I finally made up my mind when my friend Mardie talked about a recent telephone conversation with her mother. Big deal you say? Well it was years since I was able to hear on a regular phone and now Mardie, who had a severe hearing loss all her life, could chat with her mother and other family members all thanks to her new cochlear implant. She gave me all the details—the vertigo and nausea after surgery (most people do not have this problem), the early days when the sound of newspaper pages being turned was almost painful, and good stuff such as talking on the phone and listening to the news and music on her car radio. If she could do it, so could I.

It took a while to convince my HMO to approve the surgery but after that things went fast with several visits to Hopkins for hearing tests before the operation, making sure the hearing nerve was alive and well, and a visit with a psychologist to be sure I had reasonable expectations. The surgery took about 90 minutes. I went home as soon as I woke up from the anesthesia. I had no problems after the surgery and a month later I went back to get the external processor and to have the implant programmed. It was very exciting when the implant was activated—I started to hear. At first it was just noise but within minutes I could make out words and identify sounds. As we drove away from the hospital I heard the ambulance siren before I saw the flashing lights and my husband said that was when he decided that this thing might actually work. He laughed when I asked about a strange sound and told me it was the windshield wipers. I had forgotten what they sounded like.

Learning to hear again was a big adventure. Every day I would identify new sounds. Until then I had no idea that the microwave beeped and the clothes dryer made a noise when it finished a cycle. Appliances did not communicate back in the old days when I could hear. I walked around the house and garden listening to different sounds - it was wonderful. I borrowed books from the library along with the same book on tape and listened while I read the book. After a few weeks I could understand some tapes without the book depending on how clearly the narrator spoke. Some CI people understand speech right away and others may take several months. I was somewhere in the middle. It was a great moment when I stood in my kitchen and realized that I could actually follow most of the discussion on the TV in the adjacent family room.

It's been nearly ten years since my CI surgery. The new implants are smaller and much more powerful than mine but I am not the least bit sorry that I did not wait. I've had ten years of hearing conversations, music, the wind in the trees, birds singing, and—best of all—the voices of people I love.

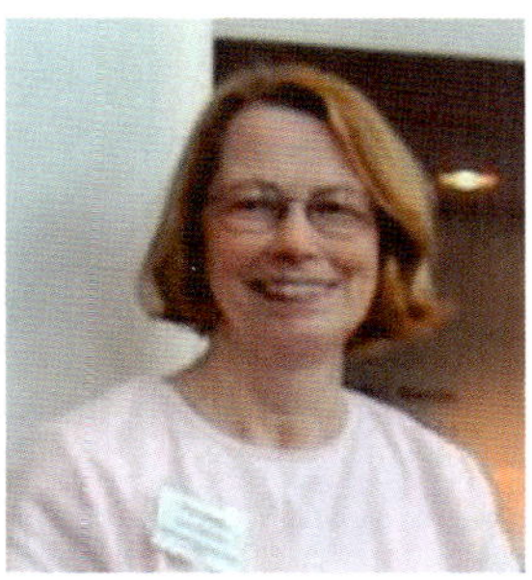

***Joan Cassidy** has been actively advocating for deaf and hard of hearing people in Loudoun County for 20 years. As an Outreach Specialist for NVRC, she works closely with Loudoun's seniors. A native of Yorkshire, England, Joan went to high school in South Africa, married an American, and has been living in the States for 45 years. She started to lose her hearing as a teenager and became deaf in her forties. She's well known for her Knitted Dolls, loves long sea voyages, and is an avid fan of PBS and BBC America.*

On Going Deaf

I've lost a sense. Why should I care?
Searching myself I find a spare.
I keep that sixth sense in repair
And deftly set it, like a snare.

Anne Stevenson

Reprinted with permission from ALDA Reader 1999

Chapter Four
Connections
Vignettes that Connect Our Lives . . .

Stressful Listening

By Cathy Kovacs

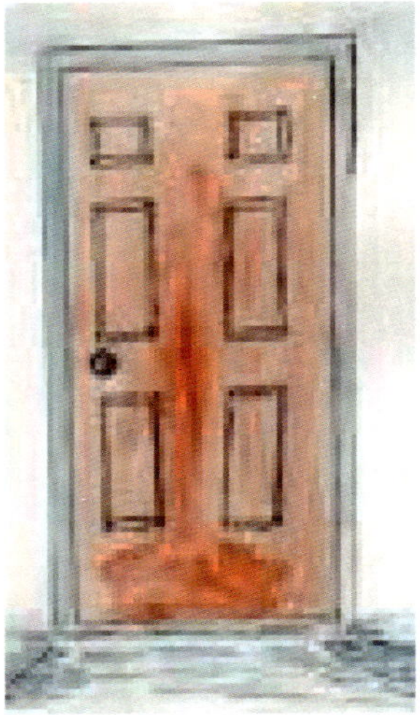

Someone slams the door—I jump, startled.

I'm at a party or with a group and the hum of people talking grows louder and louder. It gets uncomfortable—I might leave.

After a lengthy conversation, I learn someone has been telling me about their garden while I've been discussing bargains.

Everyone is listening to someone tell a joke; suddenly everyone bursts into laughter except me. I didn't hear the punch line.

I'm introduced to a pipe-smoking stranger or a person with a mustache—my heart sinks at the thought that I might not understand him or be able to read his lips.

I think I heard my name and someone saying something to me, but I was concentrating on something else and may not know where the sound was coming from. Then the speaker shouts the request again, irritated that I haven't responded, causing me to feel startled and embarrassed.

Yes—I wish people would understand how I feel. I wish someone would clue me in to the topic of conversation, especially when I go on about something unrelated! I wish someone would repeat or tell me the punch line, avoid slamming the door, remove the pipe from his mouth, get my attention before speaking.

I want to be involved in the life around me but sometimes the failures are too many so I decide to stop trying.

Communication becomes exhausting and "more trouble than it's worth," "not worth the effort," "too embarrassing," or "too dangerous a situation to not hear well."

Reprinted with permission from ALDA Reader 2007

Deafness ~ The Bubble

By Elaine Keener

I am not alone in a cave. That would be comfortable and easy.

I am in a group of people. They see me. They think I am a part of the gathering.
They do not see that I am encased in a bubble.

If, I do NOT speak
They think I have no personality,
No ideas,
No imagination.
They think I am dull,
Boring,
Stupid
They wonder why I am there contributing nothing.

If, I DO speak,
I hear two out of ten words.
I catch a word and say something,
trying to be a part of the group,
Everyone laughs or rolls their eyes,
Apparently I just repeated what was said or close to it,
I am off the target,
I ruined the flow of the conversation,
And
They think I have no personality,
No ideas,
No imagination
They think I am dull,
Boring,
Stupid
They wonder why I am there contributing nothing.

Being in the bubble,
Being seen but not connecting,
Being left out
Hurts.

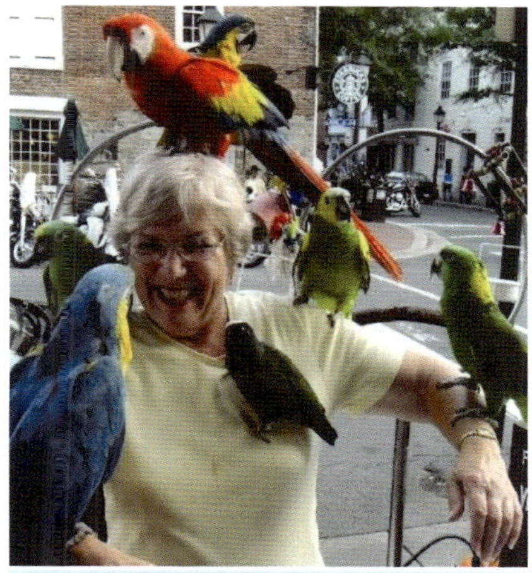

***Elaine Keener** has her Masters in Art Therapy and worked as an art therapist until 1998, when her hearing deficiency worsened to the point she could no longer hear the often whispered comments of people in therapy sessions. Realizing she was missing this important personal patient information and thereby not being as effective as she wished to be, she retired. She met with many audiologists and finally obtained a hearing aid with which she struggles to this day. Her writing tells it all.*

Many deaf people become more and more silent to save face.
But they are still cut off.

I'm going to try to connect. If I miss the gist of the conversation, I'm sorry.

90 Years Old and Deaf!

By Harriet Frankel

When I meet new people and tell them my age they always ask me what is my secret. I answer that my secret is that my mom missed turning 100 by two months. Sometimes they tell me that I don't talk like a deaf person and I explain that I'm one of many late-deafened adults who had to learn a whole set of new rules to get along in a hearing world.

If this new friend wants to know more about how I have adjusted to being deaf, which by the way, is a continuing process, I am always delighted to explain. I just love to talk because then I don't have to try to figure out what they are saying to me or fake that I have read their lips correctly and know what they are talking about.

I am like one of those survivors on a reality TV show, only I don't have to eat cockroaches or let a snake wrap around me. I just have to figure out how to live in a world without any sounds to guide me. The simple things that I took for granted before I lost my hearing now present daily problems. I still drive my car but I can't hear someone tooting his horn so I watch my rear view mirrors constantly. I don't hear my car tell me that my door is not fully closed. The world is full of sounds that warn of a problem. I don't hear sirens, I don't hear a police whistle, I don't hear my smoke alarm, I don't hear warning cries or yells.

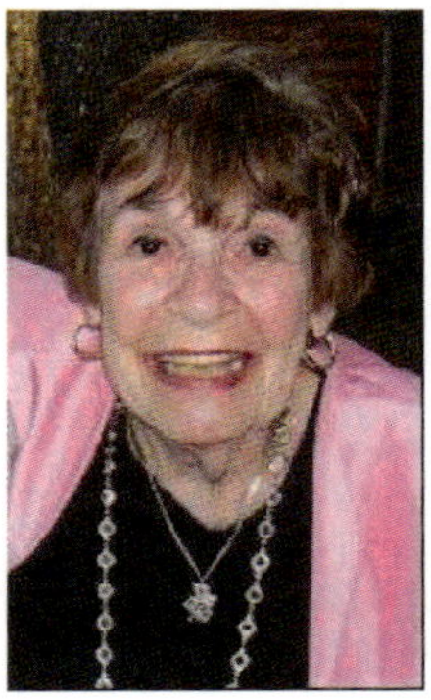

I've left the water running in my sink and flooded the apartment below me because I didn't hear the water running. Watch, watch, check, check. I now have trouble catching an elevator because I can no longer hear the ding that says which one of the bank of elevators is going up. I've learned to station myself where I can see all the lights at the same time.

But in a way, all this is a blessing. How can that be, you say? Now I must be continually alert and thinking ahead. I can't relax and be a helpless old lady but must exercise my brain at all times and we know that everyone is told to exercise, exercise! I still can smell smoke, for instance. I still can see an ambulance coming. I still can feel if I've hurt myself. I still can enjoy a hug. My mind is still working.

I want to enjoy my life while I'm alive because in my secret self, I'm still 21 years old. My knees don't agree. My hair, my teeth, my body, all know the truth, but a beautiful day is still enjoyable. I love being with my friends and family and going places. I drive with friends to play duplicate bridge around the Southeast. Last year I rode a mule halfway down the Grand Canyon.

Yes, I have to plan ahead. I see others who have overcome problems much worse than mine and they inspire me to set a good example of what people can do. I'm a survivor in a world of reality. Who knows, I may even make it to 100. If I can do it, so can you!

***Harriet Frankel** was born in Chicago but grew up in Indianapolis. She attended art school and worked as an artist in an advertising agency and had a small ad agency of her own. She celebrated her 90th birthday last year with four parties and five cakes. Harriet has been a neighborhood activist and now is active in ALDA-Peach. She continues her life despite being deaf because she loves being with people and manages with lip reading (and paper and pencil, if necessary).*

Reprinted with permission from ALDA Reader 2007

This is Not...

By Dana Gellis

This is not
The poem about my hearing loss
that I promised I'd write

Losing my hearing happened behind my back
when I wasn't listening

Why this fascination with exploring the sensual through impaired senses?

When I sit to write
I think of
The calla lilies just planted in my garden
The way the soil packs itself under my fingernails
The way the ink bleeds in a crumpled note from an old lover

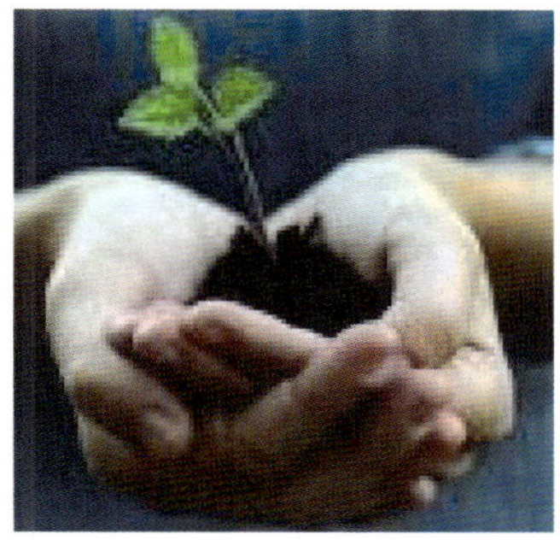

The way a ripe mango slips from my hands
and oozes its seduction down my arm
before I can suck in its sweetness
How it won't allow itself to be eaten neatly

The way my daughter's eyes tell me she's scared, or sure, or lying
The way my husband's hands are at once the most
demanding and the most healing touch I've ever felt
How he rips through my ego and loves me

I don't think about
The phone that flashes but doesn't ring for me
The doorbell that doesn't disturb me with its chime
The fire alarm that leaves me to burn quietly
The kettle that fills my kitchen with steam but never whistles
The birds that flutter and stare but don't sing
The wind that plays with my hair but never howls
Or how my pen does not make that scratching sound
that I imagine it should as it empties itself onto the page

How does one write about that which exists only in someone else's world?

***Dana Gellis** is a writer, learning consultant and teacher of the deaf. Dana grew up with a progressive hearing loss and is a recent cochlear implant recipient. As a hearing impaired individual, a professional in the field, and a parent of a hearing impaired child, Dana's experience with hearing loss is intimate and diverse. Rather than focusing on what is lost through not hearing, Dana's focus remains on the richness and beauty of life through all the senses. She also loves hiking, yoga, and gardening.*

Reprinted with permission from ALDA Reader 2007

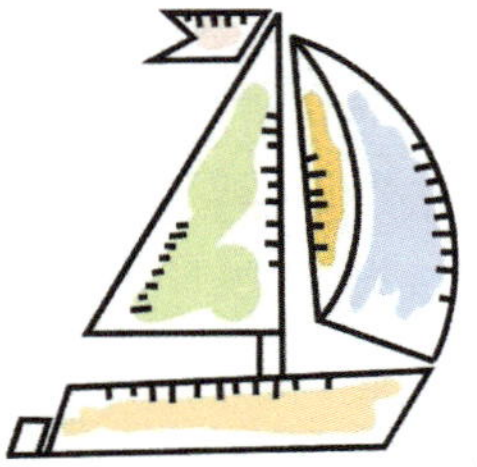

Sharing the Same Boat

By Laine Waggoner

Married for 41 years to the same man with whom I have quite an open communication style, I have probably encountered fewer problems in gaining cooperation for my special communication needs than many wives. Rex knew about my loss since we began dating. Maintaining our sense of humor and a positive attitude has been the key to the success of our relationship. It's just the two of us in this boat.

Sharing information is important. Because I know that Rex and anyone else I encounter is not a mind reader, I must explain what I am experiencing and what are my communication needs. As my "hearing-partner-in-training," he readily shares his own feelings and observations with me. This is because he has been extremely receptive to whatever new information and insights I gain and he is *very* supportive. The actor in him frequently says: "Hearing Loss is **not** a solo act—it takes a huge supporting cast."

Rex admits that during our early years together his strongest emotions were: occasional loneliness/isolation, sadness over some loss of intimacy and the reduction in the *quantity and quality* of communication, in spontaneity or sharing funny asides.

The biggest joint loss for us has been the almost complete lack of live theater, which had been a big part of our youth. Even with assistive listening devices, I still have huge speech discrimination problems. We have compensated for that by cultivating our love of film and using captioned TV and videos exclusively.

We maintain the *quality* of communication by having "dining out dates" where we can sit quietly and face one another. Rex jokes that he marvels at how I am uncannily able to detect him saying from another room, "You wanna go out to eat?"

Rex worried when I started withdrawing from some social activities because of the background noise. So it was a relief for us both when I discovered assistive listening devices about 20 years ago. My first ALD was a PockeTalker which I used for several years. Later I had a wireless FM system which worked well in restaurants and other places where I participated in group discussions. They made socializing immensely easier and less stressful.

My hearing loss has progressed to the severe/profound level. Struggling to understand conversations just keeps getting more and more tiring. Rex appreciates that...because I told him so and he is quite observant. It's comforting to know he is in my boat with me.

Laine Waggoner, MA, MS. *For the past 15 years, Laine's clients have been predominantly older adults for whom understanding hearing loss and using hearing aids is a new challenge. Laine's crusade is to help them deal effectively with the challenges of hearing loss so they will stay involved and get the most out of life. Her major interest is the physical, emotional and social impact of acquired hearing loss. In addition to earning degrees in communication and counseling, she is a Certified Hearing Loss Support Specialist and Peer Mentor in Palm Springs, CA.*

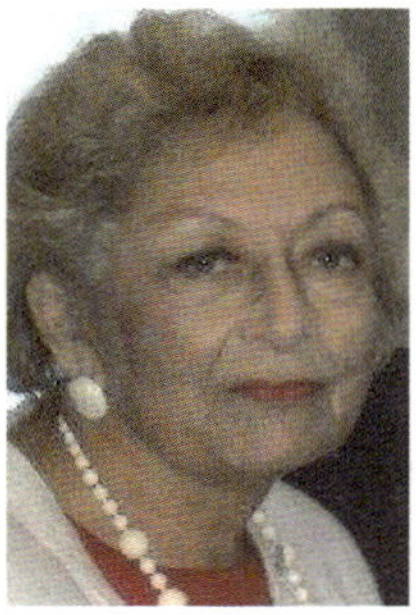

The Queen of Paradox (or Not...)

By Judy Cohen

Every day I hope that I will wake up from this cacophony of sounds and find aural order and understanding. Every day I lose just a little bit more of my ability to process sounds. Every day reality shifts and I must navigate in what seems to be an increasingly unfamiliar world.

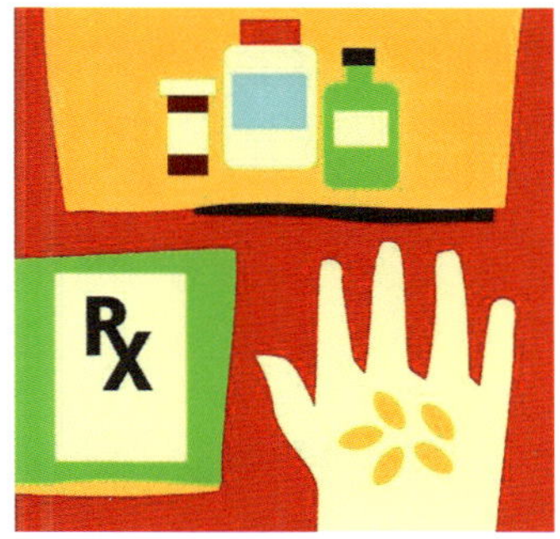

Almost a decade ago, I was diagnosed with ovarian and endometrial cancers. (The universe was having a sale: two for the price of one! Who could resist such a bargain?) When my oncologist told me that the particular chemotherapy treatment that would work best at combating my cancer also held the possibility of deafness, my response was immediate. “Dead and deaf sound the same to me.” I meant that literally as well as psychologically. Now living in the land of the “near deaf/dead,” I am shocked by my earlier assumption. Losing my hearing has sensitized me more than I could have imagined.

I make my living by listening to people. I have been a licensed psychotherapist for almost 30 years and a personal and professional coach for the last decade. I specialize in communication issues. Although I may not be able to hear, I am an expert listener. Having had the luxury of primarily relying upon my ears to hear others for most of my life, this relatively swift change of gears is teaching me now to listen through my eyes, my skin and, most importantly, my gut.

Becoming increasingly deaf has provided me with an opportunity to stop. The only way I can successfully hear others is to stop moving, stop the chatter in my mind and to fully focus my attention on the person talking to me. Deafness is my meditation room and my daily practice is to stop and focus.

In that moment of stopping and focusing, everything is available. It is the antidote to death and loneliness. Who would have thought that deafness could actually bring one to life? Cancer nearly killed me but deafness constantly forces me to be reborn one moment at a time.

***Judy Cohen, CPCC, MCC, LCSW**. Judy Cohen lives in Northern California. In the past year, her hearing has declined precipitously. Never one to miss an opportunity to make meaning out of challenging circumstances, she hopes to continue to make deafness consonant with her life.*

Reprinted with permission from ALDA Reader 2007

Accept and Adapt

By Norma Svedosh

I am a 63 year-old social worker (M.S.W., Ph.D.) who experienced late onset hearing loss. I have been wearing hearing aids for the last seven years. I am a great example of a person who was in denial, and it probably took me about five years before I admitted to having a hearing loss. As I look back over those years in denial, I became quite adept at fooling myself about my declining hearing.

As the mother of four sons, I became quite proficient during their early years at ignoring or blocking out the constant noises generated by these boisterous kids and two large dogs. It was very easy when my hearing started to diminish to claim that my hearing was fine and that I was just demonstrating the great "blocking out" skill I had developed when they were young.

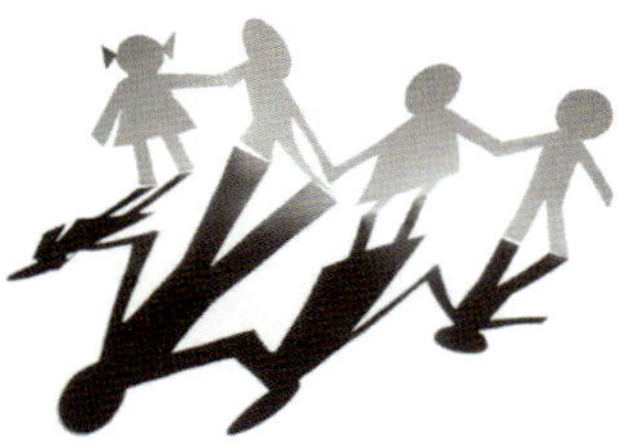

I finally acknowledged that I had a hearing problem because of two separate situations. I have six young grandchildren, and it became quite evident when I was driving them that I couldn't hear them from the back seat, particularly the higher pitched girls' voices. It upset me to realize that they probably thought that I wasn't interested enough to continue their conversations.

During this same time period, my 90 year old father was experiencing severe hearing loss. He was completely in denial, and he was having increasing difficulty carrying on conversations with family and friends. As I tried to deal with his refusal to accept his hearing loss, I realized that I was just following along the same path. Once I was fit with binaural hearing aids, my hearing difficulties diminished. Unfortunately, I was never able to convince my father to try hearing aids or other assistive devices.

Adapting to the hearing loss did not occur instantly. My first pair of hearing aids was the small, almost invisible type—CICs, because I couldn't handle the thought that they would be obvious. After about a year of using these, I finally recognized and accepted that they were not providing the functionality that I needed. I made the transition to the larger BTEs (behind the ear), which work so much more effectively for my type of hearing loss.

The hearing aids have been invaluable in helping me hear better and feel more at ease in all kinds of social situations. I also use a PockeTalker, which is a great, little handheld device that functions as a portable amplifier. My grandkids love to use it when I am driving them around. They each take turns "interviewing" me through the device from the back seat, and they think that it is so much fun to pretend that we are on TV. If I am in a noisy restaurant with friends, I just pass the PockeTalker around and never have a problem being involved in the conversation.

I am currently able to spend a lot of time enjoying my grandchildren and my friends and these experiences have been greatly enhanced because I was able to accept and adapt to my late onset hearing loss.

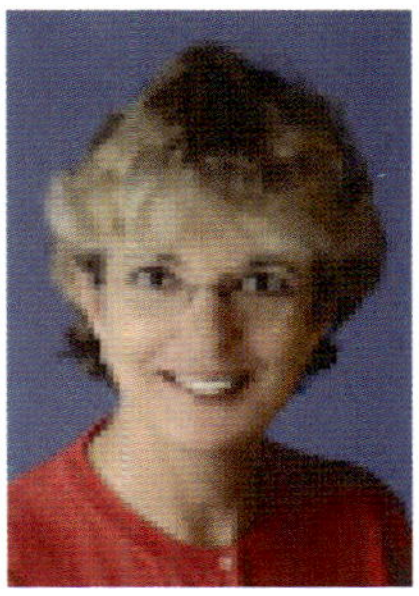

Norma Svedosh, MSW, Ph.D. *Norma received M.S.W. and Ph.D. degrees from Rutgers University. She is a licensed social worker and professional coach with a special interest in issues relating to hearing impairment due to her own late onset of hearing loss. She is a graduate of the Gallaudet University two-year Peer Mentor Certification Program, and has obtained a certificate in Hearing Loss Support from the American Academy of Hearing Loss Support Specialists at the Hearing Loss Association of America.*

File it Away

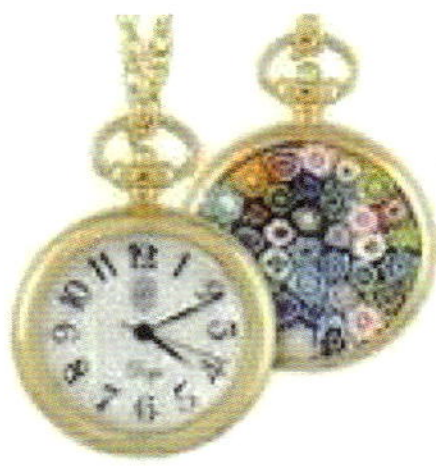

By Liz Thompson

How long ago has it been?
I can barely remember when
We could talk in the dark,
Quiet and soft,
Without having problems listening.

How long ago has it been?
Since I listened without struggling?
Or since you spoke from the heart
Without having to start
Over and over again?

How long ago has it been?
Too many years in between
And the memories fade
Of an easy day
Of hearing without any strain.

How long ago has it been?
I cannot remember when,
So I'll let the thoughts fade
And allow them to rest in the shade.
It's history, so I'll file it away.

Liz Thompson. *January 14, 1997 – As time passed, I began to accept that my hearing might really leave me completely. Realizing that one of my senses might diminish to zip was very difficult to accept! But writing has always put my thoughts into perspective. While I wrote this poem, I was actually surprised as the words hit the page! I realized I had been mouthing them prior to this time by saying, "It's okay. I'm okay. Don't worry about me. I'm handling my hearing loss just fine." I was beginning to reach a healthy state of mind, and I was growing excited about the possibilities ahead of me in the future.*

Reprinted with permission from ALDA Reader 1999

Chapter Five
Getting by with a Little Help from Friends

Support Groups
Essential for People with Hearing Loss!

By Joan Cassidy

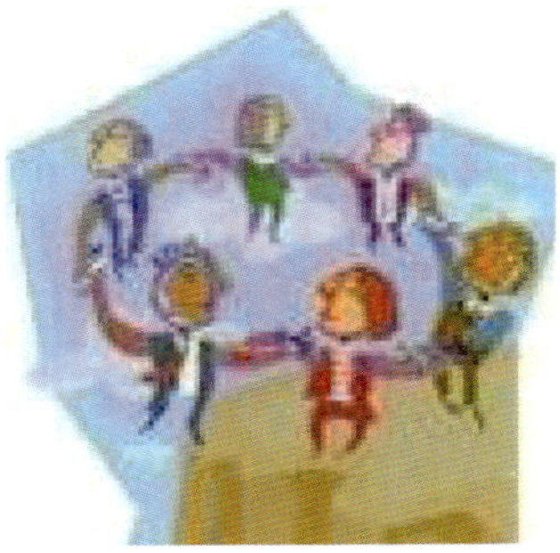

1988 was a very good year for me though it did not start out that way. It was obvious that my pact with Fate had not gone the way I wanted. My progressive hearing loss started when I was a teenager and I sort of bargained in my head "okay I'll be deaf one day but please not until I'm an old lady." Well, now I was in my forties and essentially already deaf. I got all my information through my eyes and if I could not see your face I would not even know you were talking let alone understand what you were saying. I was depressed and scared about the future because I had already lost so much—no more movies, theater, radio, TV, large parties, telephone conversations, discussion groups and more. I depended too much on my husband; I know he was worried about how I would cope if he was not there.

In May of 1988, a new friend, Betty Wiley, took me to the grand opening of the Fairfax Resource Center for the Hearing Impaired, now the Northern Virginia Resource Center for Deaf and Hard of Hearing Persons. I did not want to go because I thought I would make a fool of myself and not be able to understand what anyone had to say. Silly me, almost everyone there had a hearing loss themselves and they made sure that I could follow what was happening. I tried the assistive listening system and could hear almost every word of the speeches. It was like I got my brain back as I realized that I was as competent as anyone else if I was able to hear what was said.

The Center is where I learned about other devices such as a TTY so I could make my own phone calls and a caption decoder so that once again I could watch TV and be included in what was going on in the world. But best of all, I met other people with a hearing loss and realized that I would never again have to be alone. Even when my hearing disappeared completely I would still have friends.

The Nova One chapter of Self Help for Hard of Hearing meets at the Center and I went to some of their meetings. They encouraged me to start a SHHH group in Loudoun County where I live. SHHH is now the Hearing Loss Association of America (HLAA).

The first meeting of SHHH Nova West was in September 1988. We were a diverse group, all ages and different degrees of hearing loss, but we learned together and supported each other in any way we could. We often had guest speakers and even hosted some community awareness events ourselves, but sometimes we just talked about our problems. It was so good to share our grief and anger at losing our hearing with people who understood, rather than burdening our families with a problem they could not solve. Knowing that it would help others empowered us to acknowledge our hearing loss, speak up for ourselves and ask for help if needed. My hearing got worse but my life got better, much better. I now had friends who understood and I also had a goal—to help other people cope with their hearing loss.

A few years later I learned about another group called ALDA (Association of Late Deafened Adults) which started in Chicago in 1987. The members are people who became deaf after years of living with normal hearing. I was intrigued that they used a form of captioning for their meetings, typing out the conversation on a computer. As my hearing got worse I knew a time would come when I would not benefit from a listening system and captioning seemed the way to go.

Cheryl Heppner, director of NVRC, was already a member of ALDA so she helped organize the chapter that now meets at the Center. We call ourselves ALDA Potomac because our members come from Maryland and DC as well as Virginia. The unofficial motto of ALDA is "whatever works" and you can see this in action at our meetings. You will see some of us using sign language with a wide range of skill. One person may be writing notes, someone else typing on a computer and we all use speech reading, mime or anything we can think of to get the point across. Some of us have hearing aids or cochlear implants that help us hear each other as well as benefit from the room's assistive listening system. Nobody minds repeating a comment as many times as it takes or finding a different way of saying something. We find ways to make it work.

Like HLAA, ALDA has an annual convention, meeting at a different city each year. In 1999 our chapter hosted the convention at a hotel in Alexandria, Virginia. Hundreds of late-deafened people, friends and family members attended workshops, exhibits and special events. ALDA tends to be less educational and more of a social group than HLAA— probably because it can be harder for late-deafened people to socialize in the hearing world. For example, our March meeting is a potluck lunch to celebrate St. Patrick's Day, the fall is Oktoberfest and December is party time.

I'm still a member of HLAA because I strongly support its national goal "make hearing loss visible" and I love to get its magazine. Sad to say, our Nova West group disbanded after 13 years due to a serious case of leadership burnout. However, I just could not give it up entirely so some of us meet informally at our local Senior Center. No newsletter, formal speakers or agendas but just a good way to share our problems and solutions and simply be there for each other.

People who have a hearing loss are the real experts. We know that there is a life after hearing loss and the best place to find it is in a support group.

The Many Moods of Hearing Loss

*By Scott J. Bally, Ph.D., *PWHL*

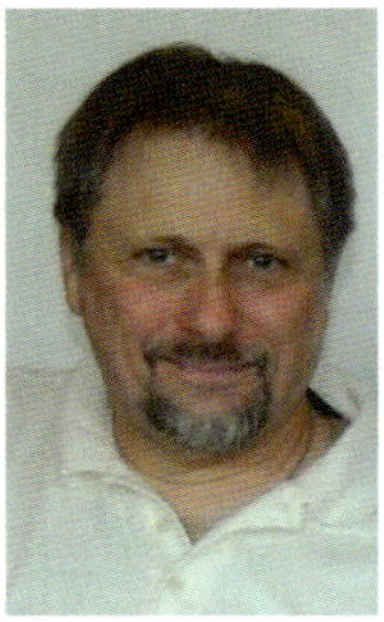

Hearing loss affects each of us differently and is a natural part of aging for many people. Understanding the various ways it might make us feel goes a long way in helping us cope with these feelings. Some folks are philosophical and comment that the golden years "seem a bit tarnished" while others take it in stride. Bette Midler said "After 40, the body has a mind of its own!" The positive thing about hearing loss when compared to other age-related conditions is that there is a **lot** you can do about it.

Many people have a deep sense of loss when hearing begins to fade. This is not unlike the loss of a loved one, our childhood home or a special relationship. After all, hearing is what connects us to others, so losing it can be pretty challenging for us. Knowing that we are experiencing loss may help us understand when we feel frustrated, angry or depressed. It's a natural way for people to respond. Many of these feelings can be alleviated when we begin to develop strategies that reconnect us with others. Knowing we are not alone in these feelings can give us a sense of normalcy and assure us that we are not the only ones who have ever felt this way.

Sometimes our loved ones are aware that we have a hearing loss before we know it. They notice that we say "huh?" or "what?" more often, misunderstand the things they say and generally talk more loudly. When hearing loss occurs gradually over a long period of time in our lives, we often do not notice these changes in our behavior. Sometimes, in an effort to help, others will point out that we might think about having a hearing test. Usually this is done out of kindness and concern…and a desire to communicate with us more easily because they care about us.

Our first response may be to challenge the suggestion because there is still a stigma about hearing loss (we are less "competent"). However, when we let it percolate for awhile, the realization will usually manifest itself that we, indeed, do need some help.

Research shows that the average person waits seven years between realizing he or she has a hearing loss and actually doing something about it. Imagine!

Another point to consider is that those who love us are experiencing similar feelings to ours. We are so focused on how hearing loss affects us that we don't think about how it affects others. For every frustrated listener, there is a frustrated talker; for every isolated listener, there is an isolated talker...you get the point.

Sharing our hearing loss-related feelings with others who have hearing loss can be very uplifting. It helps us understand these feelings better and gives us hope that there are solutions and a brighter tomorrow.

***Scott J. Bally, Ph.D., CCC-SLP** sits on the faculty of both the speech-language pathology and audiology programs in the Department of Hearing, Speech and Language Sciences at Gallaudet University and teaches in both master's and Au.D. programs. He holds a B.S. in education from Truman State University, an M.S. in communication disorders from Colorado State University, and an M.S.W. from Gallaudet University. Dr. Bally earned his interdisciplinary doctorate in gerontological aural rehabilitation from the Union Institute.*

*Person With Hearing Loss

Do you Read Lips ?

By Bonnie O'Leary

You try! Did you know that only 30 percent of the English language is visible on the lips? In other words, 70 percent is not! Hearing people often assume that hard of hearing people are fluent lipreaders. That is a myth, but we can improve our skills over time.

We call it "speechreading," because we have to observe the speakers' lips, teeth, tongue, facial expressions, gestures, rate of speech, accent, and pitch of voice. That's a lot to pay attention to at once! Every speaker has his or her own unique facial architecture and vocal tone, which is why it can be so easy to speechread one person and impossible to speechread another.

English has many sounds that look the same on the lips, such as "p/b/m," "f/v," or "t/d/l/n." We call these sounds "visemes." Learning to speechread involves being able to identify the different visemes in the context of conversation. It also requires the use of numerous strategies, such as asking the speaker to repeat, rephrase, give us key words, or even spell a word. It also involves understanding what we can control such as where we position ourselves in relation to the speaker, turning up the lights, turning down the music, asking the speaker to move to a quieter room with us, and so on.

There are many factors that determine how successfully we can speechread in any given conversation. These include background noise, lighting, objects that could block our view of the speaker, our degree of hearing loss and how long we've had it, the diction of the speaker, or how we're feeling that day. Familiarity with the topic is important too; it might be easier to speechread "I had a great time on my vacation" than "hey, how do you spell cyclooctanedicarboxaldehyde?"

Next time someone says "you can hear when you want to," let them know what your challenges are!

Listening with Both Eyes

By Jeanne Murray

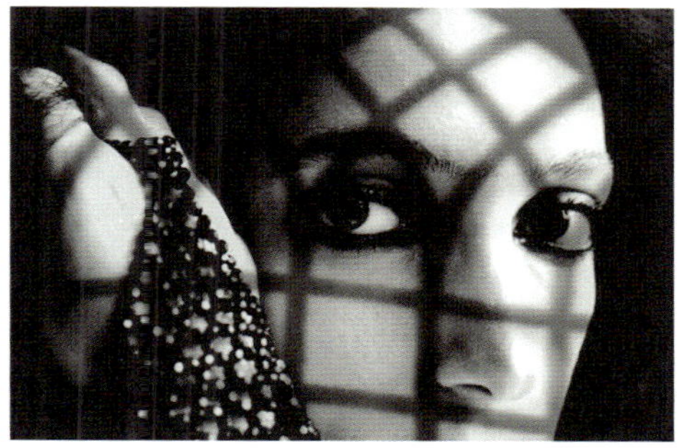

When talking with you
there's something I do,
it makes some nervous;
I hope not you.
I'll read your lips
for the words you send.
Hearing is something
I cannot pretend.
I think by doing this,
I hear more than most;
because on your face
is the very place
the story will show.
I see so much happiness
with the smiles that glow.
Also, the sadness
when the sorrow flows.
I see fear
if it is near,
cause it is with my eyes
that I do hear.
So, pardon me
if I stare.
I'm reading the words
you are sending to share.

Reprinted with permission from
ALDA Reader 2005

The Invisible Condition

Common Misconceptions About Hearing Loss and Aging

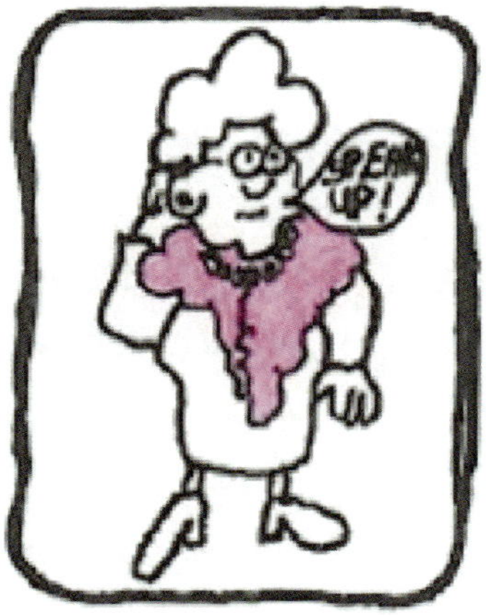

"WHY DON'T YOU SPEAK UP?"
"YOU YOUNG PEOPLE ALL MUMBLE THESE DAYS"

Hearing loss in older people may begin gradually and progress slowly. In early stages, it is often unrecognized.

"SHE HEARS WHEN SHE WANTS TO"

There is often inconsistent listening behavior. This is because the parts of hearing which are important to speech (the high frequencies) usually deteriorate sooner than those which relate more to environmental sounds (low frequencies).

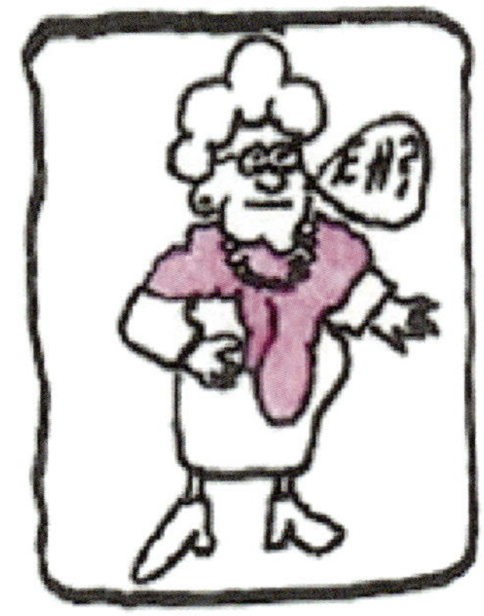

"I HEARD, BUT I DIDN'T UNDERSTAND"

"ALL RIGHT! THERE'S NO NEED TO SHOUT!"

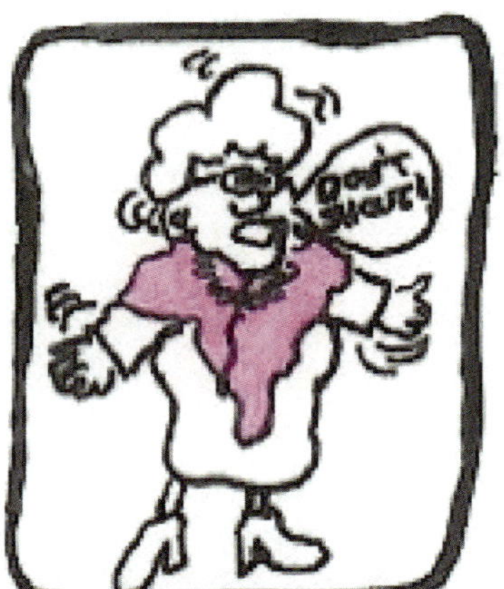

There may also be problems of distortion. This can be like trying to listen on a bad phone line. Making it louder does not always make it clearer.

"WHY ON EARTH DON'T THEY GET A HEARING AID?" ("...and stop being a bother to me)"

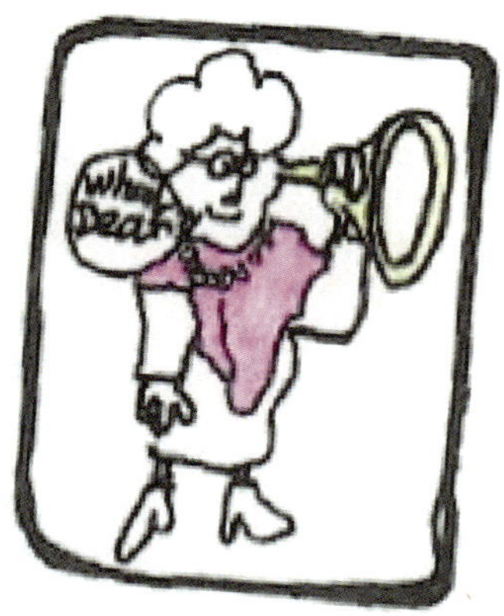

A well-fitted hearing aid can be a great help. However, hearing aids make sound louder. They do not "correct" hearing. Even the best aid remains on the outside. The person's own defective hearing system must still take the message between his or her EARS and his or her BRAIN. The brain must then decode (understand) the imperfect message which has arrived there.

Patience and understanding are needed. COMMUNICATION IS TWO-WAY! Your understanding and appropriate management can make a difference.

Reprinted with permission from the Hearing Loss Association of America

The Invisible Condition

Tips for Talking With Hard of Hearing People

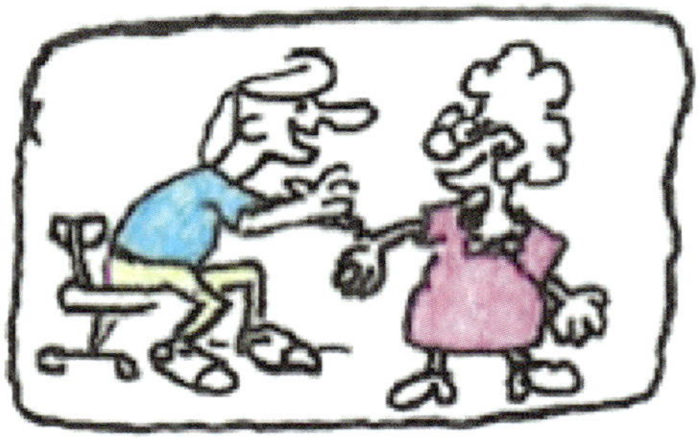

Gain attention. Face the hard of hearing person directly and on the same level whenever possible.

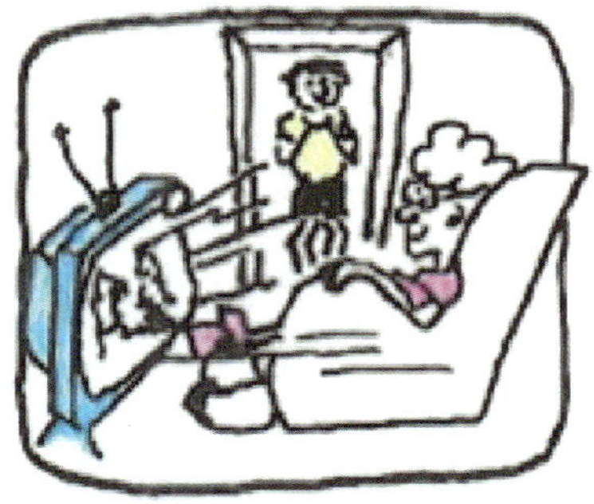

Avoid background noise. Turn off or turn down the TV or radio. Do not talk from another room.

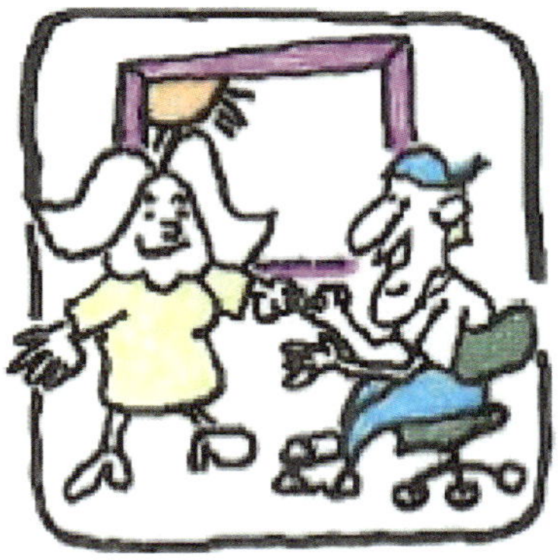

Be careful that the light is on your face, not behind you. Hard of hearing people need to see you clearly to help them to understand.

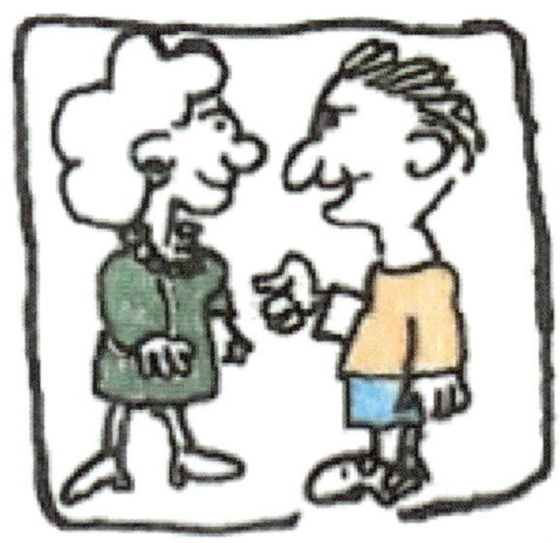

Speak normally—if anything, a little slower. Don't exaggerate lip movements. Don't shout.

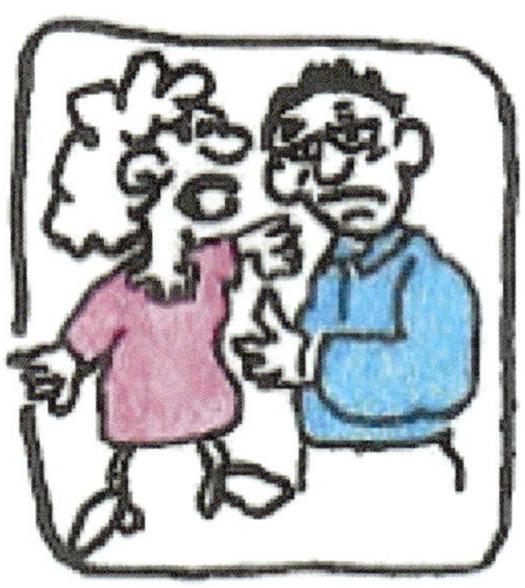

Get to the point. If you are not being understood, say the same thing in different words. If necessary, write it down.

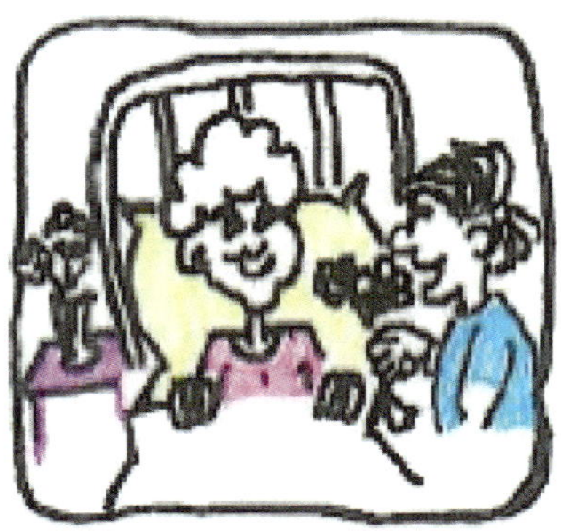

Understand that hard of hearing people manage less well when they are tired or ill. Even with the best hearing aid, a person may have difficulty understanding speech.

Home for the Holidays

By Scott J. Bally, Ph.D.

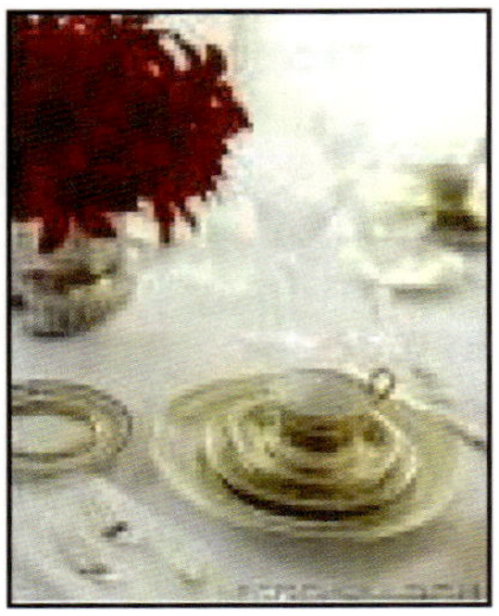

When holiday seasons approach, the anxiety level of many individuals with hearing loss may begin to increase. It's those holiday gatherings that put fear in our hearts. Have faith! Here are some of the best, tried and true coping strategies that can make your season brighter:

Isolate conversations

You may anticipate speaking to many different members of your family or social circle, especially your favorites. However, you already know that communicating in a noisy living room or family room may be difficult, if not frustrating.

Seek out a more isolated area for your conversations such as a den, breakfast nook or sunroom. Invite people you'd like to chat with to join you. "It's so good to see you. I've been dying to hear about your new job. Let's go into the den so I won't miss a single word."

Give yourself a break. We all know that communicating when you have a hearing loss to contend with is tiring under the best of conditions...and it can be exhausting in the worst. When you feel yourself reaching your limits, give yourself permission to take a break. Take a walk around the block. Find an empty bedroom and lay down for ten minutes. You'll find yourself refreshed and ready to face the next round of conversation.

Choose your dinner partner

To the extent possible, identify individuals with whom you have an easy time communicating. It might be someone like an uncle with a deeper voice, a cousin who enunciates clearly and is easy to speechread, or a friend who remembers to use communication strategies which help you. Don't hesitate to ask someone to sit with you. If you know the seating assignments will have been pre-arranged, contact your host or hostess in advance, give a brief explanation, and ask to be seated next to your desired dining companion.

Guide the dinner table conversation. Being careful not to completely dominate the conversation; ask people about things you already know something about. For example, if a family member or friends may have already told you about a forthcoming trip that has since occurred, ask about their journey. Even if you already know some of the details, there is bound to be a new thought or observation and you may ask for an update. Speechreading in familiar territory puts you at a significant advantage.

Ask closed-set questions

Another strategy that may be used is to ask "closed set questions." If you ask a general question such as "Will you tell me about your trip?", there are a multitude of answers that might be forthcoming. However, if you ask, "What cities did you visit?" it helps to limit the answers to the names of the cities. This "closed set" is usually much easier to lipread.

Buffets are better

They are better because you may be able to choose a cozy corner to eat in with one, maybe two other people. You might ask your host if it's okay to go into the den or another small room. However, if it is a sit-down dinner, you should probably try to make the best of it. Don't frustrate yourself by trying to follow conversations that ricochet around the table. Try to engage the people to your right, left and across the table individually in one-on-one conversations.

Again, select known topics or those that may not matter much if you miss parts of what was said. Try to get your "best visiting" done either before or after the meal. And, if understanding during the meal becomes frustrating, simply focus on enjoying the bounty of the food before you.

Be the family historian

A number of years ago, a woman I'll call Aunt Janet shared her "secret to success." She designated herself as the "family historian." Before large family gatherings, she would contact various family units and invite them to bring photographs and stories for the family scrapbook. She would set up shop in a small room with a card table and several chairs. She would have the family album open on a table, ready to share the pictures and stories she had already collected, and, pen and glue stick in hand, be ready to add the latest contributions.

Small family groups would take turns sitting with Aunt Janet and giving her updates. Each of the younger children would offer at least one picture and explain what it was all about ("Here I am with my soccer trophy." "This is Farley, the new family dog.") Aunt Janet would use a glue stick to put it in place on their family units' page and write the information under it on the page. Janet commented that she felt she always knew more about her family than anyone else and she had a deep feeling of belonging and worth in her self-appointed role.

Explore technology

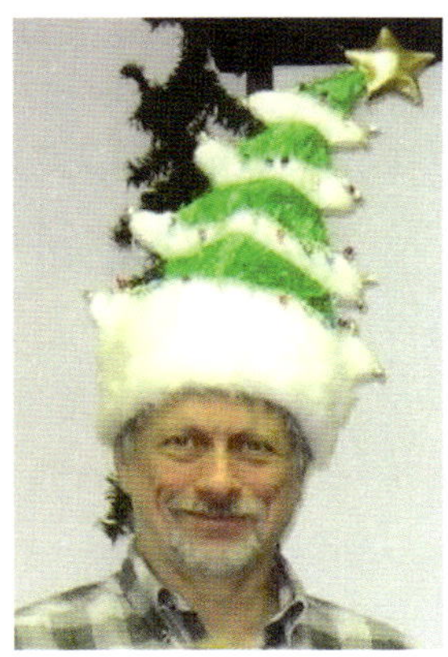

Preparing for a family gathering may be a good time to review hearing technology. There are some useful technologies that work especially well in such group situations. Both directional and hand-held microphones, for example, will bring the speaker's voice closer while eliminating some of the background noise.

Conference microphones which you place on the dining table may be less useful when many people are talking at the same time and table noise such as clinking glasses and silverware will be able to be transmitted. View these events as great opportunities to try new technologies to see if they'll work for you.

What Caregivers Should Know

By Gay Nagy

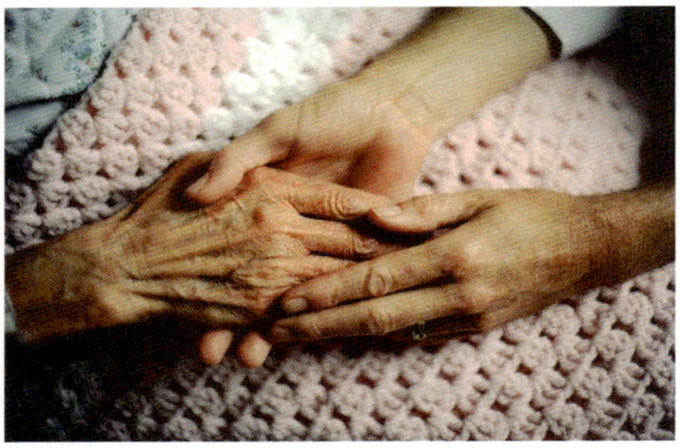

Caring for a person who is hard of hearing can be a daunting experience because communicating becomes such a challenge.

Just because someone wears a hearing aid does not mean that he or she hears normally. Often, the person *can hear but cannot understand* what's being said.

Here are some helpful hints to ease frustration for both the caregiver and the person with hearing loss:

When you are speaking:

- Be sure you have the listener's attention
- Face the person—do not speak with your back turned or from another room
- Speak slowly and clearly
- Do not chew gum or food while you are speaking
- Keep objects, such as fingers and pencils, away from your mouth and face
- If you have a mustache, keep it trimmed above your upper lip
- Be patient and smile
- Be aware that saying "never mind," "forget it," or "I'll tell you later" is hurtful
- Keep a pad and pen nearby for writing messages back and forth
- Offer clues to accompany your words, such as gesturing, pointing or miming
- Use picture cards to point to what you mean when other strategies fail

Assess the hard of hearing listener:

- How is the person feeling today? Well? In pain? Fatigued? Anxious?
- Has he or she started on different medication that could affect hearing, energy level, or ability to focus?
- Does the person have vision problems that could affect the ability to lipread?
- Can the person insert hearing aid batteries without help?
- Are the batteries in the hearing aid and are they charged?

How is the listening environment?

- Be sure there is no background noise, such as TV, radio, or noise from another room
- Ensure that the overall lighting is good
- Avoid a light source behind the person speaking
- Keep the room at a comfortable temperature
- Remove objects such as flower arrangements, candles, or centerpieces blocking the person's view of the speaker
- Stay within a 3-to-6 foot proximity of the person to facilitate lipreading
- Make use of a PA system or listening system when needed

Think about what you're saying:

- Does the listener understand the topic and know what's being discussed?
- Is the vocabulary familiar?
- Is the listener apprised when the subject is changed?
- Can you use key words or rephrase the message?

In general:

- Keep extra hearing aid batteries in a recloseable, plastic bag along with instructions on how to replace the batteries and a copy of the business card of the person's audiologist
- Keep a set of instructions in another recloseable, plastic bag on how to assist the person with use of his or her hearing aid(s), cochlear implant or other devices
- Be sure that other caregivers, family members or supervisors know where the person keeps his or her hearing aids when they are not being worn

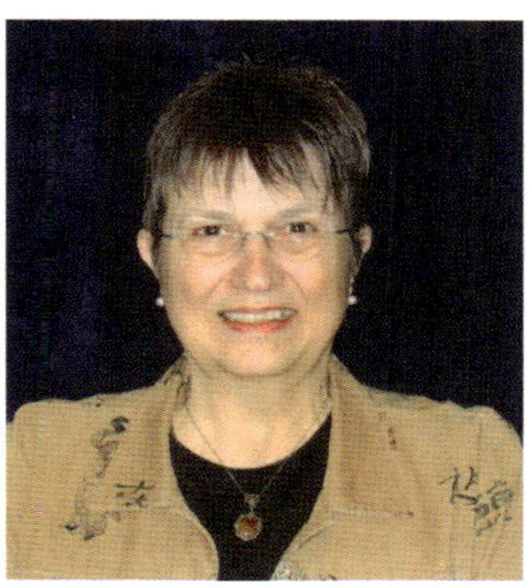

***Gay Nagy** holds a B.S. in Elementary Education and Speech Therapy from Northern State University in South Dakota. In her 19 years at NVRC, she worked with the community on many aspects of hearing loss, using her personal experiences with hearing loss as a basis for her programs. She is fluent in sign language. Gay provided staff trainings to businesses and agencies, as well as presentations on hearing health and coping strategies to consumers and families. Gay's public relations work included staffing exhibits at numerous community events. She retired in January, 2009.*

From Riches to Remnants to Richness

A Southerner's Tale of Surviving Hearing Loss in the Workplace

By Homer Mullins, J.D.

Somewhere during the late summer months of 2000, amidst all the hustle and bustle in the halls and back offices of a large international, Atlanta-based law firm where I was a litigator, I found myself musing numerous vexations.

- Why don't our hotshot young lawyers speak up and look me in the eye when talking so I can understand them?
- Why do my colleagues walk away in the middle of my answer to a question they just asked me?
- Why do they no longer drop by for small talk or invite me along for lunch or a drink after work?
- Why do people seem to prefer communicating with me through my secretary about matters concerning firm business?
- Why can't I remember the names of firm colleagues I've known for years and see in the hall almost every day?
- Why am I forever feeing utterly exhausted?
- Why all of a sudden and for the first time in my professional life is the quality and timely completion of my assignments being called into question?
- Why am I feeling worthless and abandoned at work, and unloved at home?
- And finally, why am I consumed with the fear that I'm going to be fired?

If you're reading this article, you might recognize at least some of my puzzlements as being those of a person gripped by a significant, undiagnosed late onset hearing loss. My case was complicated by the presence of an Auditory Processing Disorder (APD) which served to exacerbate the symptoms of an otherwise mild case of ADHD for which I have well compensated all my adult life. If you detected signs of depression and anxiety, you were exactly right, both being driven primarily by feelings of helplessness and loss of control over what was happening to me. Would my career survive it and, if forced to find another livelihood, what could I do to continue supporting my family in a respectable life style and get my kids through college? Once the depression settled in, I felt totally unmotivated, unable to get out of bed and get started on...anything. For the immediate term, I decided that by continuing work in such a state, I could unwittingly make things much worse for myself and my clients, not to mention the possibility of increasing the risk of loss to myself and the firm for malpractice claims and possible professional sanctions.

So, I took a six-month paid medical leave.

The turning point for me came after finding an expert audiologic diagnostician at the University of Florida. He was able to diagnose my condition as a moderate to profound, mixed unilateral hearing loss, accompanied by an APD. He also gave me his opinion as to the likely cause of the constellation of symptoms I was experiencing: the confluence of these disorders was exacerbating the impact of each one on the other so that the totality of the effect was much higher than either of them acting alone. During his wrap-up he suggested that I "might want to be looking for something else to do."

After leaving his office, I felt a tremendous sense of relief. I felt liberated from the fear of ignorance as to the nature of my condition and where it was taking me. Most important, I knew that I could no longer practice law in any form that would satisfy me. I also believed that the prospects of my competing successfully in the academic world for another advanced degree promised to be highly stressful.

I decided that my ideal career would be one I could comfortably learn within a reasonable period. To mitigate any feelings of having been relegated to second class citizenship, it was vital to me that I find work I truly believed was important, had the potential of providing me with a reasonable income given the circumstances, and was likely to make a positive difference in the life of someone else.

It struck me that in addition to having the experience of a 30-year practicing attorney, I was already something of an expert in the fields of hearing impairment and APD. Plus, and perhaps most important, I had become aware through personal experience, how serious and insidious were the problems of auditory dysfunction as they impacted a challenged person's ability to understand speech. In a profession where complete understanding of speech is critical to adequate representation of and advocacy for a client's position, I couldn't imagine anything I could do that would be more important.

Since, as far as I can determine, I'm alone and first-ever in this field as to lawyers, it was up to me to prepare myself as best I could for performing the role I was seeking to play. The first big break came when I was selected for the Peer Mentor for the Hearing Impaired Program at Gallaudet University which I have now completed. It has provided me with a solid background from which to operate. I was also fortunate to have met and formed several partnerships—"Odyssey Hearing Solutions" and "The Legal Ear" with Norma Svedosh, a Ph.D. social worker, also hearing impaired, whom I met in a training program to become ADHD coaches. We both graduated from that program and have since become credentialed as Senior Certified ADHD Coaches.

When I started four years ago, the typical service I would offer would be to lawyers who were struggling to cope with the same sort of issues with which I had dealt, i.e., cognitive issues brought on by auditory and attention dysfunctions which were threatening their ability to remain competitive in a field where they are measured by standards set by the unimpaired. I quickly learned there were other areas in the law firm context where my help could be of significant value:

- Consulting with the firms' HR and Lawyer Recruiting Departments on matters of accommodation for disabled employees or any special requirements for recruiting programs for hearing impaired lawyer candidates under the Americans with Disabilities Act
- Consulting with firms on the appropriate handling of lawyers under the State Bar's Rules of Professional Conduct that management suspects to have significant hearing issues, especially where that lawyer is in denial of the problem and refuses to seek help
- Consulting with firms to set up a program to ensure that its lawyers are practicing in full compliance with the Rules on an on-going basis

Lawyers must be educated to the fact that hearing loss is becoming increasingly prevalent at younger ages and is a serious problem with far-reaching civil and professional implications for lawyers and their firms, and that it's not a nuisance even if it does come with age! Once over this hurdle, most firms are very receptive to "hearing" what services you can offer them and quite willing to take the initiative toward making it safe for their lawyers to step forward for assistance when needed. A major means of providing such an environment is to promote programs designed to eliminate the stigma that makes so many unwilling even to admit to the existence of a problem.

At the risk of sounding like a "~~Pollyanna~~" "Pollyhomer," I believe I was able to survive and rally to my challenges by following the advice my Dad gave me to always be vigilant for opportunity in the face of "disappointment." Though my standard of living is not what it was, I find myself in a far more personally fulfilling and uplifting position than I've ever had. In addition, I have the satisfaction of knowing I'm carrying the message as a living example to others in my profession. Through the use of modern technology in the form of hearing aids and assistive listening devices, there's hope that lawyers challenged by hearing loss at the height of their careers can, if patient, survive the "bump" and go on to achieve their goals and serve the profession by mentoring other lawyers with similar setbacks.

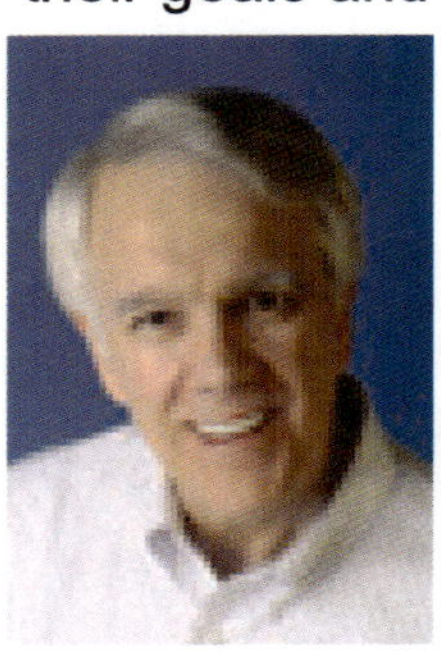

Homer S. Mullins, J.D. *Homer is a graduate of the College and Law School of Emory University. Until 2001, when he left Atlanta-based King & Spalding, he practiced law in a variety of different settings, from general counsel of a large publicly-held savings bank to JAG officer in the U.S. Air Force. Homer recently received his certification in Peer Mentoring for People with Hearing Loss from Gallaudet University and the American Academy of Hearing Loss Support Specialists.*

Hearing Dogs: True "Miracle Ears"!

By Cheryl Heppner

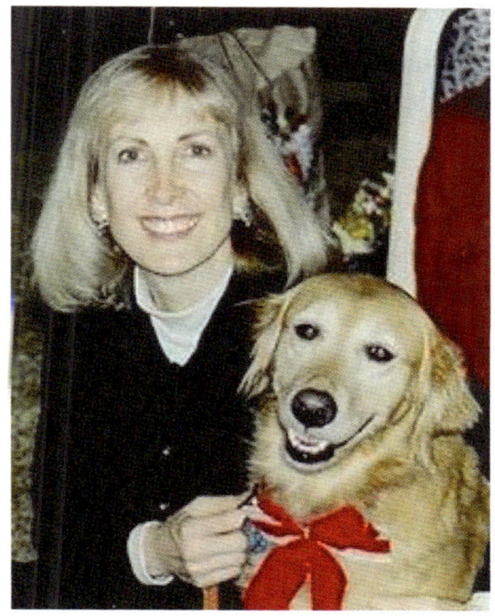

Cheryl and Dana

It had been a long, tiring day at a convention. I sat on my hotel bed, kicked off my slippers, and took out my hearing aids. I was eager to climb under the covers and read in glorious silence until I dozed off. Suddenly a reddish-golden paw pressed against my leg, and I turned to see Dana, my hearing dog, whip around and head toward the door.

I followed her and peered through the peephole but saw only an empty hallway. Puzzled and a bit annoyed by Dana's false "door knock" alert, I turned to go back to bed when Dana's paw pushed hard against my thigh, and she wheeled once again toward the door. Her body language made it clear that it was imperative for me to respond immediately.

When I cracked open the door to check for someone outside the range of the peephole, Dana pushed past me and into the hallway. There was no one in sight. I called her, but she refused to come back. As I walked toward her to grab her collar, she ran a few more feet up the hallway. Again I walked toward her and made a grab; again she ran a few more feet ahead of me.

I was becoming furious at Dana's disobedience, but my temper suddenly evaporated as I glimpsed people pouring out of other rooms, scurrying for stairways. I tried to comprehend the confusion I was seeing since I could hear nothing without my hearing aids. Then I realized that I was feeling the vibrations of many feet pounding, perhaps mixed with the vibrations from loud alarms going off as people raced to evacuate from the building. Dana's extraordinary intelligence and training saved my life; she led me out of the hotel to safety during a fire that night.

Hearing dogs like Dana, and my current dog, Galaxy, are trained to alert their human partners to sounds such as a door bell, door knock, teakettle whistle, kitchen timer, telephone ring, smoke alarm, and the various beeps and bells of kitchen and laundry appliances. They usually alert through physical contact to get the partner's attention, and then lead their partner to the sound source.

This work is very challenging. Not only is the dog expected to alert its partner to a sound even if it is tired or asleep, it must alert for the sound every time it occurs. Many other kinds of assistance dogs are given a command or encouragement to do their work. A hearing dog has to start working without any direction or motivation from its partner and follow a five-step process accurately and quickly. It must (1) recognize a sound it has been trained to alert to, (2) find its partner, (3) give the partner an alert, (4) locate where the sound is coming from, and (5) lead the partner to it. Failing to do just one step could mean that the partner will miss a phone call, visitor or pot boiling over.

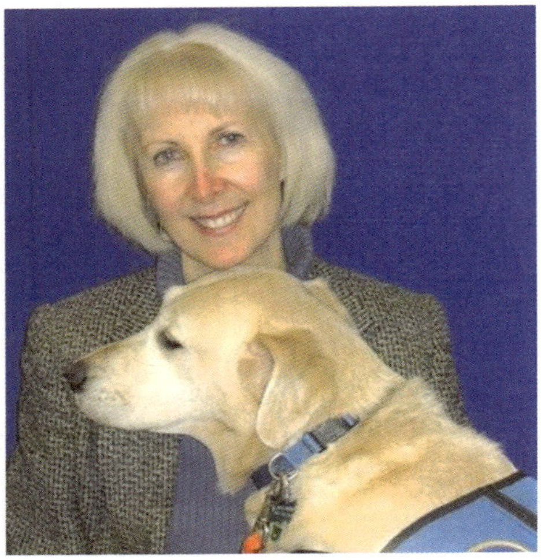

Cheryl and Galaxy

Of course there can be exceptions to the process. If Galaxy hears the smoke detector, she is trained to alert me and then lie down; this tells me that I need to immediately leave the building. Otherwise Galaxy might well be leading me in the direction of a fire. The night that Dana's actions got me to safety during the hotel fire, she used intelligent disobedience to lure me out the door and down the hallway.

As you can imagine, hearing dogs must possess qualities beyond good health and intelligence. They must have a work ethic so strong that they are self-motivated and enjoy working. They must have a good temperament, be friendly and adaptable. They must be able to pay attention, respond to commands, and remain under control even when they are startled by distractions such as cars or buses backfiring, children hitting them, or other pets attacking them.

Hearing dogs come in all shapes and sizes. Many people prefer to have smaller hearing dogs because there's less to bathe, groom, feed, and pick up after. Smaller dogs also fit more easily under restaurant tables or airplane seats. Dana, who passed away of old age in 2005, was a Golden Retriever. Galaxy, my partner since 2002, is a Labrador/Golden Retriever cross.

I've experienced challenges in having a hearing dog, too. These include a loss of anonymity because my dog attracts a lot of attention in public, and occasional confrontations with people who don't realize the ADA assures right of access in public places to service dogs. Also, regardless of how busy my schedule is or how bad the weather, attending to my hearing dog's needs is a 24/7 responsibility.

But these challenges are small compared to the one that was toughest by far, facing and accepting the time I would have to say goodbye to a partner. That will never, ever get easier.

Having a hearing dog is one of life's greatest joys. The relationship is built on love and trust, and the dog quickly learns your idiosyncrasies and quirks, your moods and feelings. A dog can bring great comfort when you need a friend, providing true "pet therapy." And after the day's hard work, there is a lot of time for playing with favorite toys, for special long walks, for running and chasing, and relaxation.

A Treasure Trove of Resources!

Come on down! We'd love to have you visit us.

Here are some of the popular services we provide:

One-on-one mentoring – Not sure whether to get a hearing aid? Not happy with the one you have? How about challenges you might be having trying to communicate with your family and friends? Spend time with one of our staff who will give you information to help you make wise choices for your situation.

Personalized information – What would you like to know more about – cochlear implants? Restaurant strategies for people who are hard of hearing? Factors affecting speechreading? We have 21 free facts sheets on a variety of topics relating to hearing loss that might help you.

Assistive listening device demonstrations – Would you like to try out a TV listening system? How about making a call on one of our amplified phones so you can test the volume? You can also see how a flashing alert system works and try out a personal amplifier in the privacy of our device demonstration room.

Technology Assistance Program (TAP) and Loan to Own (L2O) - Pages 31 and 32 provide the details about TAP and L2O; all you have to do is make an appointment with Debbie Jones and come try the various devices available through these programs.

Web site – www.nvrc.org – Want to visit us from the comfort of your home? Our website is open 24 hours a day, 7 days a week, and you can easily contact us with your questions through info@nvrc.org. We usually respond within a few hours.

Community Center – Would you like to attend a program or support group at NVRC? Our all-access meeting room offers a state-of-the-art induction loop system, FM receivers, and CART (captioning) for programs. Refreshments are provided, and this is a great opportunity to meet other people who have hearing loss.

Daily e-mail news – Would you like to receive the latest information on deafness and hearing loss from around the world? Sign up for our free email news service by contacting cheppner@nvrc.org.

Just remember – there is hope and help at NVRC!

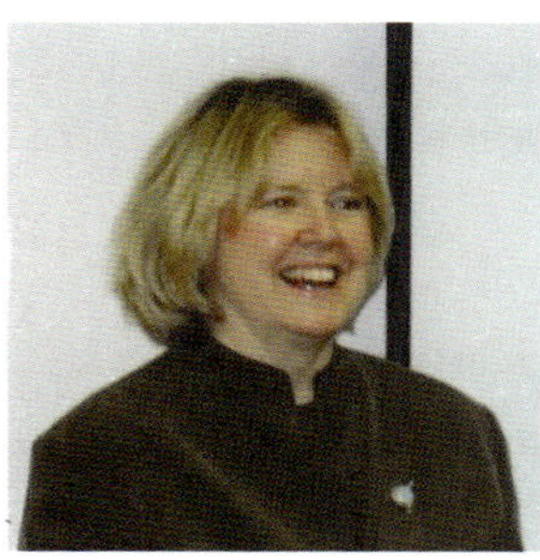

***Melody Hotek** joined the NVRC staff in 2004 as Director of Operations after working as a volunteer and serving on the NVRC Board of Directors. Her background is in administration with more than 30 years experience in supervisory positions and a degree in Health Care Administration. She oversees the web site, newsletters, meeting room, volunteers and the planning and implementation of NVRC's major events. Melody is our go-to person for graphics and problem solving.*

Peering into the Future

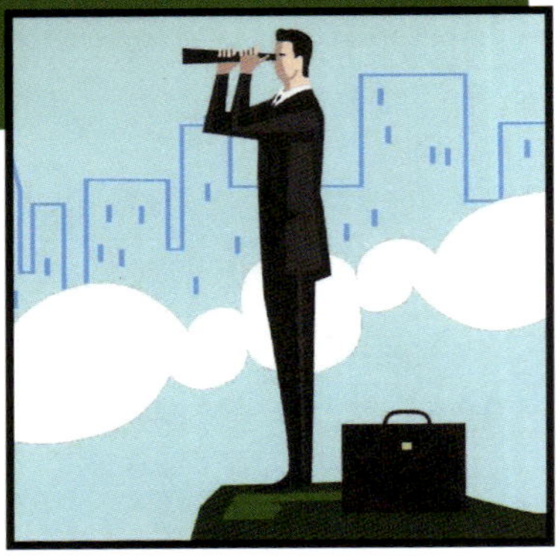

If we were to describe all the research that's under way to help hearing loss and all the technologies that are being developed we'd have to write another booklet!

Here are three that are getting a lot of attention at the moment.

Hair cell regeneration

Did you know that birds, fish and amphibians don't go deaf? When the hair cells in their hearing mechanisms die off, they naturally regenerate. Scientists are hopeful that stem cell-based research will unlock the mysteries of the genetic program for hair cell regeneration in humans. Although some success in treating deafened guinea pigs and chickens in laboratory experiments has been reported with cautious optimism, testing in humans is still a few decades away. But scientists are encouraged by the possibilities!

Captioned radio

How's that?! How on earth can you caption a radio? It works a lot like close captioning does for television. A data stream is piggy-backed onto the standard audio signal. The text can then be read on a radio fitted with a display. The system will only work with digital broadcasts, but Internet-based solutions are being developed. Soon you will be able to tune your computer to the radio station and read what is being spoken on your monitor! Not only that, you'll be able to select the size, type and color of the font that is easiest for you to read!

Implantable magnetic nanoparticles

A company called NanoBioMagnetics, Inc. (NBMI) has been conducting research on laboratory animals that involves implanting nanoparticles in the middle ear that respond to a magnetic field. This operates on a similar principle to the electromagnetic hearing aid, but the difference is that the device is very small and surgically implanted in the middle ear. In March, 2008, NBMI received the patent to commercialize the product, and we are waiting to hear about further developments in the marketplace.

Additional Resources

Assistive Listening/Alerting Devices

Harris Communications
15155 Technology Drive
Eden Prairie, MN 55344
1-800-825-6758
www.harriscomm.com

HEAR-MORE
42 Executive Blvd.
Farmingdale, NY 11735
1-800-881-4327
www.hearmore.com

Cochlear Implants

Johns Hopkins Hospital
Dept. of Otolaryngology
601 N. Caroline Street
Baltimore, MD 21287
410-955-1080
www.hopkinsmedicine.org

University of Virginia
Cochlear Implant Program
PO Box 800871
Charlottesville, VA 22908
434-982-0129
www.healthsystem.virginia.edu

Speech & Hearing Centers

Gallaudet University
Hearing and Speech Center
800 Florida Avenue NE
Washington, DC 20002
202-651-7328
www.gallaudet.edu

George Washington University
Dept. of Speech & Hearing Sciences
2115 G. Street, NW
Monroe Hall of Government
Washington, DC 20052
202-994-7362
www.gwu.edu

Hearing Aids

Hearing Planet, Inc.
100 Westwood Pl., Suite 300
Brentwood, TN 37027
1-800-432-7669
www.hearingplanet.com

Hearing Dogs

Canine Companions for Independence
286 Middle Island Road
Medford, NY 11763
631-561-0200
www.cci.org

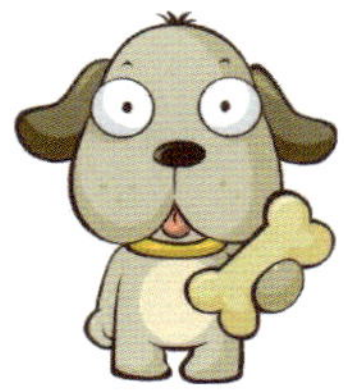

Fidos for Freedom
PO Box 5508
Laurel, MD 20726
410-880-4178
www.fidosforfreedom.org

International Hearing Dogs, Inc.
5901 East 89th Avenue
Henderson, CO 80640
303-287-3277
www.ihdi.org

General Hearing Loss Information

National Institute on Deafness and
Other Communication Disorders
31 Center Drive
Bethesda, MD 20892
301-496-7243
www.ncid.nih.gov

Tinnitus

University of Maryland Medical Center
22 S. Green Street
Baltimore, MD 21287
410-328-5947
Tinnitus-Hyperacusis@smail.umaryland.edu

Support Groups

Association of Late-Deafened Adults (ALDA) www.alda.org
RD1@alda.org

Hearing Loss Association of America
National Headquarters
7910 Woodmont Avenue
Bethesda, MD 20814
301-657-2248
www.hearingloss.org

Hearing Loss Association of America
Northern Virginia Chapter
3951 Pender Drive, Suite 130
Fairfax, VA 22030
703-352-9055 ext. 106
info@nvrc.org

Say What Club
www.saywhatclub.com
info@saywhatclub.com

NVRC maintains a database of more than 2,000 resource and referral listings. The few we have included here have been given good reviews by the members and friends of NVRC who have used them.

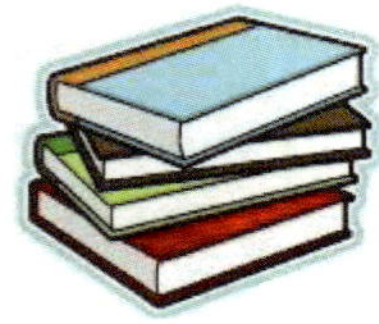

Books

Chelsea, The Story of a Signal Dog
Paul Ogden
Available in many book stores

Living with Hearing Loss
Marcia Dugan
Gallaudet University Press
www.gupress.gallaudet.edu
1-800-621-2736

Ototoxic Drugs Exposed
Neil G. Bauman, Ph.D.
Center for Hearing Loss Help
49 Piston Court
Stewartstown, PA 17263
717-993-8555
info@hearinglosshelp.com

Speechreading, A Way to Improve Understanding
Harriet Kaplan, Scott Bally, Carol Garrettson
Gallaudet University Press
www.gupress.gallaudet.edu
1-800-621-2736

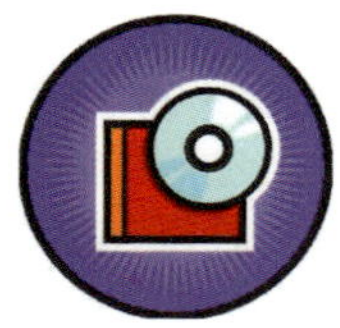

DVD with Manual

I See What You Say
Self-help Lipreading Program
Hearing Visions
3427 Sequoia St.
San Luis Obispo, CA 93401
805-546-0442
hearngvisions@yahoo.com

Acknowledgements

From the moment it was just an idea, "I Can't Hear You!" involved the enthusiasm and energy of many people, either directly or peripherally.

NVRC would like to thank Christine Seymour, President of ALDA, Inc., for giving us permission to reprint so many touching poems, cartoons and personal stories from various ALDA publications. We would like to acknowledge the ALDA authors for whom we had no contact information and therefore no photo or bio: Anne Stevenson, Liz Thompson, Cathy Kovacs, and Jeanne Murray. We also thank Toni Barrient of HLAA's national office in Bethesda, MD, for providing "The Invisible Condition" cartoon.

Our sincere appreciation also goes to Gallaudet University's Peer Mentor program graduates, Homer Mullins and Norma Svedosh of Princeton, NJ, and Laine Waggoner of Palm Springs, CA, for writing their stories specifically for this publication. Other contributors who donated their time are Dana Gumb of Alexandria, VA; Lenore Benderly of Longboat Key, FL; Lise Hamlin of HLAA in Bethesda, MD; Dr. Neil Bauman of Stewartstown, PA; and Dr. Scott Bally of Bethesda, MD. We thank them all for so willingly finding the time to write new material amid their torturous schedules.

Special thanks to friends of NVRC who graciously reviewed this publication and offered invaluable comments and suggestions: Terri Lynch, Director of Arlington's Agency on Aging; Patty Butler-Burkhart, Director of Resident Services, Goodwin House, Alexandria; Cheryl Johnson, Countywide Director of Senior Services, Arlington County Senior Adult Programs; Brenda Cox, Arlington Commission on Aging; Jim and Barbara Morris of Arlington; Grace Starbird, Director of Fairfax County's Area Agency on Aging; Jeff Hotek of Grossberg Company CPAs; Fran Barker; Natalie Kerr, Delaware Hospice (Ret.); and Lita Arnold.

We also thank our cadre of senior readers/reviewers who made many wonderful suggestions: Anne Meagher, Betty Beale, Else Elliott, Fran McComb, Dana Gumb, Helen Bishop, Neil Cassidy, Elizabeth Clement, Ona Mathers, Edwin Palmer, Bob Timmons, and Mary Beth Spink.

An extra special thanks to audiologist Leslie Lesner, M.A., for reviewing pages three through 18 for factual accuracy. And to our Editor-in-Chief, Marianne Confalone, much appreciation for an outstanding job. You're the cat's meow!

Most importantly, NVRC would like to thank Mike DeFries and his daughters, Diane and Vicki, who were involved in the progress of the booklet from conception to completion. We thank Mike in particular for his guidance, editorial expertise, patience and good humor. Thanks also to Liala Merzadazada for cooking so many delicious lunches for our editorial meetings by the lake (with Mike's special Borscht!). And in our hearts, we thank Grace Abelson DeFries, who was the inspiration for the booklet. NVRC is honored to have been entrusted with this project.

My Personal Information

Name: ____

Ear, Nose & Throat Doctor (ENT)

Name:

Address:

Phone:

Audiologist/Dispenser

Name:

Address:

Phone:

Hearing Aid

Make/Model:

Year Purchased:

Batteries

Battery Size (number/color):

Notes

2996780

Made in the USA